EMERGENCY CARE AND TRANSPORTATION

OF THE
SICK AND
INJURED

STUDENT REVIEW MANUAL

Exercises for the EMT-A and EMT-I

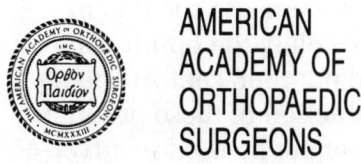

AMERICAN
ACADEMY OF
ORTHOPAEDIC
SURGEONS

CREDITS

American Academy of Orthopaedic Surgeons Board of Directors, 1993

Bernard A. Rineberg, MD
Bernard F. Morrey, MD
James W. Strickland, MD
Joseph A. Buckwalter, MD
Howard P. Hogshead, MD
John B. McGinty, MD
Augusto Sarmiento, MD
Robert N. Hensinger, MD
Robert D. D'Ambrosia, MD
James H. Beaty, MD
Marc F. Swiontkowski, MD
James G. Buchholz, MD
Gene E. Swanson, MD
William C. Collins, MD
Douglas W. Jackson, MD
Barry P. Simmons, MD
Thomas C. Nelson, *ex officio*

First Edition

Copyright © 1994 by American Academy of Orthopaedic Surgeons

All rights reserved. No part of the *Student Review Manual* may be reproduced, stored in a retrieval system, or transmitted, in any form, or by any means, electronic, mechanical, photocopying, recording, or otherwise, without prior written permission of the publisher. Address requests to American Academy of Orthopaedic Surgeons, 6300 N. River Rd., Rosemont, IL 60018. Telephone: 1-800-626-6726

ISBN 0-89203-083-6

Library of Congress Catalog Card Number 93-73963

Published and distributed by: American Academy of Orthopaedic Surgeons

10 9 8 7 6 5 4 3 2

Staff

Executive Director: Thomas C. Nelson
Deputy Executive Director: Fred V. Featherstone, MD
Director, Division of Education: Mark W. Wieting
Director, Department of Publications: Marilyn L. Fox, PhD
Senior Editor: Lynne Roby Shindoll
Production Manager: Loraine Edwalds
Assistant Production Manager: Kathy M. Brouillette
Editorial Assistants: Susan Baim, Kathryn M. O'Brien

The material presented in the *Student Review Manual* has been made available by the American Academy of Orthopaedic Surgeons for educational purposes only. This material is not intended to present the only, or necessarily best, methods or procedures for the medical situations discussed, but rather is intended to represent an approach, view, statement, or opinion of the author(s) or producer(s), which may be helpful to others who face similar situations.

Some drugs and medical devices demonstrated in Academy courses or described in Academy print or electronic publications have FDA clearance for use for specific purposes or for use only in restricted research settings. The FDA has stated that it is the responsibility of the physician to determine the FDA status of each drug or device he or she wishes to use in clinical practice, and to use the products with appropriate patient consent and in compliance with applicable law.

Furthermore, any statements about commercial products are solely the opinion(s) of the author(s) and do not represent Academy endorsement or evaluation of these products. These statements may not be used in advertising or for any commercial purpose.

ACKNOWLEDGMENTS

Medical Editors

David G. Lewallen, MD
Mayo Clinic
Rochester, Minnesota

Lynn A. Crosby, MD
Creighton University
  School of Medicine
Omaha, Nebraska

Principal Authors

Michael G. Smith, REMT-P
Director of Paramedic Training
Tacoma Community College
Tacoma, Washington
Paramedic, Shepard Ambulance
Seattle, Washington

Richard W. Vomacka, BA, REMT-P
Vice President and Editorial Director
Educational Directions, Inc.
Akron, Ohio

Thomas R. Nehring
Assistant Vice President
Medcenter One
Bismarck, North Dakota

Portions of the *Student Review Manual* have been adapted from:

Reviewing Basic EMT Skills: A Guide for Self-Evaluation

Contributing Editors

Alexander M. Butman, BA, EMSI
Thomas J. Hauser, BA, EMT
Richard L. Judd, PhD, EMSI
E.L. Pendagast, Jr., MD, ACEP
Steven E. Reinberg, BA, EMSI
Bertram M. Siegel, EMSI

REVIEWERS

Our thanks to the following individuals who, throughout the development of this project, either reviewed the entire manuscript or selected chapters of the *Student Review Manual*. Their comments and suggestions were extremely helpful to the editors and authors.

Alice "Twink" Dalton, BSN, NRPM
Creighton University
Omaha, Nebraska

Joseph G. Ferko, III, MS, PhD, DO
Philadelphia College of Osteopathic Medicine
Philadelphia, Pennsylvania

Charles "Punky" Garoni, BA, EMT-P
University of Texas Health Science Center
 at San Antonio
San Antonio, Texas

Catherine T. Kelly, RN, MSN, CEN, CCRN
St. Francis Hospital Emergency Department
Poughkeepsie, New York

Peggy Linial
Des Plaines, Illinois

Mark Lockhart, NREMT-P
St. John's Mercy Medical Center
St. Louis, Missouri

James P. McGraw, RN, MN, CCRN, CEN
Harris Methodist Hospital Fort Worth
Fort Worth, Texas

CONTENTS

Chapter 1	Introduction	1
Chapter 2	Legal Responsibilities	6
Chapter 3	Personal Safety	12
Chapter 4	Basic Anatomy	22
Chapter 5	Assessing Vital Signs	30
Chapter 6	The Respiratory and Circulatory Systems	39
Chapter 7	Cardiopulmonary Resuscitation and Basic Life Support	49
Chapter 8	Airway Obstruction	67
Chapter 9	Control of Bleeding and Shock	79
Chapter 10	Wounds and Bandaging	91
Chapter 11	The Musculoskeletal System	101
Chapter 12	Fractures and Dislocations	113
Chapter 13	Spinal Injuries	130
Chapter 14	Injuries of the Head, Eyes, Mouth, and Face	143
Chapter 15	Injuries and Problems of the Chest, Abdomen, and Genitalia	157
Chapter 16	General Medical Emergencies	171
Chapter 17	Pediatric Emergencies	189
Chapter 18	Substance Abuse	199
Chapter 19	Childbirth	208
Chapter 20	Environmental Injuries	217
Chapter 21	Poisons, Stings, and Bites	234
Chapter 22	Interacting With Patients	246
Chapter 23	Crisis Intervention	255
Chapter 24	Handling and Packaging the Patient	265
Chapter 25	Ambulance Operations	275
Chapter 26	Intravenous Therapy	283
Chapter 27	Advanced Airway Management	302
Chapter 28	Defibrillation for EMTs	318
Chapter 29	Case Studies	336

Chapter 1

Introduction

Purpose of the *Student Review Manual*

As an EMT, you will provide emergency care based on the knowledge you obtain as a result of your study and training. The body of knowledge an EMT must retain encompasses a wide area, including specific facts, general concepts, and precise physical skills. All of this knowledge must be learned thoroughly and permanently so that it can be applied with confidence in the varied and difficult situations that you will encounter. It must be so familiar that it can be recalled quickly and with certainty, under pressure at a moment's notice.

Becoming familiar with this vast amount of information is not an easy task. Even after thorough study, it is often difficult to judge whether you have mastered a subject. How can you tell if you really remember all of the information you might need? How can you tell if you remember it in enough detail without misunderstanding or uncertainty?

This review manual is designed to help you evaluate your mastery of the material you learned in class and read in *Emergency Care and Transportation of the Sick and Injured*. While you need not have specifically read the textbook to answer the questions in this review manual, each and every question is referenced to the revised fifth edition of the textbook. Working through this review manual will help you to identify areas in which you need further development, whether you are a student or a practicing EMT.

If you are just entering the field, it is impossible for you to imagine all of the many difficult situations that you may encounter in the field. That is why the *Student Review Manual* includes an entire chapter of case studies to give you simply a taste of what is "out there." In this chapter and throughout the manual, you will be presented with complex questions and situations that will require you to think about hidden problems and unforeseen situations. These questions will present problems the way they appear to the practicing EMT, requiring you to consider the "big picture," rather than merely focusing on isolated problems.

The *Student Review Manual* is not an EMT textbook; it assumes that you have thoroughly studied the content, or are studying the content as you proceed through the chapters. Rather, this review manual will provide you with a way to assess what you have learned through your reading and your classroom work. To become completely comfortable with all the information presented during your training, you must answer questions, relate facts and situations, learn to anticipate problems, and be able to prioritize the steps in proper patient care. This review manual will provide you with the kind of exercises that develop a lasting and useful knowledge base for prehospital emergency care procedures.

Chapter 1

It is also hoped that this review manual will help you to begin preparing to sit for the National Registry Examination. While this review manual is not a practice examination, it does include the same type of multiple-choice questions that you are likely to see on classroom and national examinations.

Organization of the *Student Review Manual*

The *Student Review Manual* contains 29 chapters, 28 of which are made up entirely of multiple-choice questions. Each chapter includes the following elements:

1) a list of chapter goals;

2) a section of multiple-choice questions;

3) a section of answers with brief explanations of the answer;

4) a page-by-page correlation of the question/answer to the revised fifth edition of *Emergency Care and Transportation of the Sick and Injured*.

Chapter Goals

The chapter goals are knowledge, rather than skills, based and are similar to the goals in many of the chapters of the revised fifth edition of *Emergency Care and Transportation of the Sick and Injured*. The purpose of the chapter goals is to prepare you for the questions that lie ahead. You should also review the chapter goals after you have finished the questions to decide whether you feel you need additional review.

Multiple-Choice Questions

The principal function of any multiple-choice question is to directly assess knowledge, skill, or ability in a specific content area. A good multiple-choice question will not be "tricky" or ambiguous, but will be straightforward and carefully worded. A well-written multiple-choice question assesses only content that is considered important to the profession or area of study.

This review manual contains several different types of multiple-choice questions. Some of the questions only require you to recall, or recognize, the key. This type of question is called a basic knowledge question. Clearly, basic knowledge is essential to successful EMT practice. Questions that ask you to identify parts of the human body, to recognize types of injuries, or to recall specific types of equipment are very important.

However, multiple-choice questions that address higher thinking skills are particularly useful for EMTs. Although basic knowledge is certainly necessary, you will often be required to quickly organize pertinent information to make an accurate patient assessment. You must also be able to set priorities or make decisions about providing appropriate patient care in unusual and/or stressful situations. That is why this review manual contains many questions presenting complex situations and an entire chapter of case studies.

Introduction

Answers with Explanations
A separate section containing the answers with brief explanations of the answer follows the section of multiple-choice questions. These explanations focus primarily on the correct answer, or key. In most cases, the explanations will not detail why the other answer choices, or distractors, are not correct.

Correlations
Following the explanation of the answer, you will find a page-by-page correlation of the answer to the revised fifth edition of *Emergency Care and Transportation of the Sick and Injured*. As with the explanations, the correlations refer you to the area in the textbook where the correct answer is discussed.

Writing Multiple-Choice Questions

Writing effective multiple-choice questions requires great skill. Often ambiguity or other flaws in a question are not noticed until after students respond to the question. To make sure that the multiple-choice questions in this review manual are of the highest quality possible, the *Student Review Manual* has been edited and reviewed extensively by content experts with experience in teaching and writing multiple-choice questions.

The Stem
A typical multiple-choice question consists of three parts: a stem, the distractors, and the key. The stem of the multiple-choice question is the part that poses the question, problem, or situation to which you must respond. A well-constructed stem has several critical features, including: 1) a single, complete question; 2) clear, concise, accurate language; and 3) important, relevant content.

The Distractors
A multiple-choice question will present several options from which you must select the correct answer. One of the options is always the correct answer, or "key." The other, incorrect options are called distractors. Well-written distractors should be plausible, or believable, to students who do not know the key; they should be relatively short, compared with the stem; and all distractors should be about the same length as the key. The distractors should not be tricky or trivial; they should not contain negative wording; and they should not contain information that will "tip off" the key.

The Key
The key is the option that is intended as either the correct or best answer. In some instances, there may not be a single "right" answer to the problem in the question. In fact, more than one answer to the problem may exist, but is not presented in the question. However, the option indicated as the key is intended to be the best of the choices presented. In discussions with your instructors and other members of your class, other answers and related points to consider should be pursued. It is hoped that a fuller understanding of emergency medical care by all participants will be the result.

Chapter 1

Test-Taking Strategies

In the course of your EMT education, you will be preparing for and sitting for several examinations. Because examinations are often a source of anxiety, especially if you have not been in the classroom for a while, we have included a list of nine test-taking strategies to help you prepare for your next examination.

Mental Preparation

The best way to prepare for any test is with thorough studying. Keep up with class readings and set aside a regular time for study and review. Waiting until the last minute to prepare for a test often only results in confusion. You may benefit from studying and reviewing with other students.

Physical Preparation

Proper rest the night before a test is essential, as is proper nutrition. Also allow ample time for traveling to the test site, parking, and locating the test room with at least 15 minutes to spare before the start of the test.

Materials Preparation

Make sure you have all necessary materials ready, including writing materials, calculators, and scratch paper, if necessary.

Anxiety

While some anxiety actually improves test performance, some students become overwhelmed in a testing situation. Think about the test as several small pieces to complete, rather than as one massive test. This may help reduce your anxiety.

Pacing

As you begin a test, you should quickly note the time allowed, the total number of questions, and the starting time in order to pace your work. Check your progress often. For example, if there are 100 questions and you have 2 hours for the test, you will have about 1.2 minutes per question. Remember to avoid lingering over any one question for too long. Skip any troublesome question and return to it later as time permits.

Guessing

It is almost always to your advantage to respond to every test question, even to those for which you do not know the correct answer—in other words, to guess. In many cases you may be able to eliminate one or two of the answer choices right away, giving you a better chance for guessing the correct answer.

Making Notes

If your answer sheet is not machine scored, you may often be able to make notes, charts, and diagrams on your answer sheet. Blank areas in the margins can be used to jot down memory aids or to calculate the solution to a problem.

Introduction

Testing Myths
Students often have faith in the following testing myths. Following this advice is likely to result in choosing the wrong answer.

Myth 1: The longest option is usually correct.

Myth 2: When in doubt, C is usually correct.

Myth 3: An answer choice that contains "always, never, or all" cannot be correct.

Myth 4: Don't change answers: the first answer you select is usually correct.

Myth 5: Most questions contain "tricks" or "hidden" meanings.

Finishing
When you have finished the test, you should make sure you have:

1) answered all of the questions;
2) written your name on the test and/or answer sheet.

Summary

Practices in emergency care are constantly scrutinized and revised. Accepted procedures are often changed, and there are often differences from one location to the next with regard to what is proper. If anything presented in this text appears to conflict with practice you have been taught, bring it to the attention of your instructor or training director. A full discussion of differences will not only clarify any conflict but help you to gain a better understanding of the question involved.

Chapter 2

Legal Responsibilities

Chapter Goals

The exercises in this chapter are designed to help the student review:

- the laws of consent as they relate to providing patient care.

- the elements of the doctrine of negligence.

- the forms of immunity granted by law.

- records and reports for specific legal situations.

Legal Responsibilities

Multiple-Choice Questions

Select the correct answer for each of the following questions. Each question has only *one* correct or best answer.

1. An 8-year-old boy has a lacerated artery. You have tried to contact the parents, but they cannot be reached. Your next step would be to:

    A. phone the emergency department physician and ask for permission to proceed with treatment.

    B. ask the police for permission to proceed with treatment.

    C. take the boy to the emergency department but give no treatment.

    D. assume the parents would give consent for treatment.

2. The decision to begin treatment of a patient who is unconscious, or so seriously injured that his or her judgment is impaired, is based on the legal doctrine of:

    A. applied consent.

    B. conditioned consent.

    C. implied consent.

    D. replied consent.

3. A woman who has severe abdominal pain refuses to go to the hospital. Her husband asks you to transport the patient regardless of her wishes. The most appropriate course of action would be to:

    A. transport the patient because her condition warrants it.

    B. transport the patient because her husband requests it.

    C. respect the patient's wishes.

    D. explain to the husband that transport is not needed because the patient's condition is not life threatening.

American Academy of Orthopaedic Surgeons

Chapter 2

4. Good Samaritan laws are designed to protect:

    A. responders from civil damages when they stop to give emergency care, as long as they act within the bounds of their training.

    B. a person who stops at the scene of an accident, decides he or she is unable to help, and then leaves the scene.

    C. a person who stops at the scene of an accident and commits an act of gross negligence.

    D. victims of accidents from incompetent first aid treatment.

5. You stop at the scene of an accident to help an injured person, but leave before other help arrives. Failure to continue care is called:

    A. negligence.

    B. breach of duty.

    C. abandonment.

    D. malpractice.

6. Which of the following activities is a principal function of the EMT at the scene of an automobile accident?

    A. Provide "crowd control" until law enforcement officials arrive and then begin treating patient(s) with minor injuries.

    B. Obtain all necessary information about the patient(s) and the accident before leaving the scene.

    C. Pronounce a patient dead, if the patient is dead.

    D. Collect evidence for law enforcement officials before they arrive.

7. The legal doctrine of negligence consists of what three elements?

    A. Standard of care, duty, abandonment

    B. Standard of care, lack of consent, duty

    C. Duty, breach of duty, causation

    D. Duty, abandonment, lack of consent

Legal Responsibilities

8. In which of the following situations has actual consent been given?

    A. A 5-year-old child who says, "Make me better"

    B. An unconscious 26-year-old woman who has a bleeding head wound

    C. A 35-year-old man who has a slight concussion but holds his bleeding arm out for bandaging

    D. An 86-year-old man who stares blankly at his bleeding leg and says, "What happened to me?"

9. You begin treating a 4-year-old child who has second-degree burns on both legs. The burns cover the legs from the knees to the feet. The parent states that the child jumped into the bath water before it was tested for temperature. If you suspect abuse, the most appropriate action would be to:

    A. try to get the parent to confess.

    B. call law enforcement officials to the scene.

    C. treat the patient and then report your suspicion to the dispatcher.

    D. tell the parent that the patient needs treatment at the hospital and then transport the patient.

10. A local celebrity has severe injuries as a result of an automobile-truck accident. The highway is closed by law enforcement officials, but the media is allowed to cover the story. A reporter approaches you and asks the condition of the patient. You should:

    A. ignore the reporter.

    B. answer the reporter's questions as best you can.

    C. tell the reporter the patient will be fine to protect his privacy.

    D. explain that you cannot comment and that the reporter should contact the hospital.

Chapter 2

Answers

1: **D.** You should assume that the parents would give consent for treatment. (ECTSI 5, p. 22)

2: **C.** Implied consent assumes that in a true emergency an unconscious or mentally impaired patient would give consent to treatment. A true emergency is a situation in which there is a significant risk of death, disability, or deterioration of condition. (ECTSI 5, p. 22)

3: **C.** A competent patient has the right to refuse treatment. The EMT should explain to the patient why transportation to the hospital for treatment is advisable. However, the EMT in this case must respect the patient's wishes if she refuses treatment. In any case of patient refusal, the EMT should follow local protocols. (ECTSI 5, pp. 22–23)

4: **A.** Good Samaritan laws are designed to protect from civil damages those who render aid within the bounds of their training. However, these laws cannot and do not prevent suit. (ECTSI 5, p. 24)

5: **C.** Abandonment occurs when treatment is begun and then discontinued before the patient is turned over to another equally or better trained health care professional. (ECTSI 5, p. 21)

6: **B.** The EMT is responsible for collecting as much information about the patient as possible before leaving the scene. The EMT may not pronounce a patient dead. Only a medical examiner or physician has the legal authority to pronounce a patient dead. Crowd control and collection of evidence are functions of law enforcement. (ECTSI 5, pp. 26–27, 78)

7: **C.** Duty, breach of duty, and causation must all be present for the legal doctrine of negligence to be applicable. Once called to the scene, an EMT has a duty to help a victim. Failure to provide care, or providing care that is not consistent with the care that would be provided by another EMT, is breach of duty. If the breach causes further injury, then the EMT has acted in a negligent manner. (ECTSI 5, p. 20)

8: **C.** Actual consent occurs when the patient expressly authorizes you to provide care or transport to the hospital. Actual consent may take the form of words, a nod of agreement, or other expressions of approval. (ECTSI 5, p. 21)

Legal Responsibilities

9: **D.** The EMT is obligated to report cases of suspected child abuse to the proper authorities. The best course of action in this case would be to take the patient to the hospital to document the suspicion. The EMT should not attempt to obtain a confession from parents or call law enforcement officials to the scene. The dispatcher would not be considered an appropriate authority. (ECTSI 5, pp. 26, 568)

10: **D.** The EMT should not comment on the condition of any patient, except to report to the hospital or to turn the patient over to equally or better trained health care professionals. (ECTSI 5, pp. 25–26)

Chapter 3

Personal Safety

Chapter Goals

The exercises in this chapter are designed to help the student to:

- explain the importance of nutrition and physical fitness for the EMT.

- describe the hazards associated with fire.

- describe common water and ice hazards.

- identify the hazards associated with electricity, terrain, falling objects, and confined spaces.

Personal Safety

Multiple-Choice Questions

Select the correct answer for each of the following questions. Each question has only *one* correct or best answer.

1. In a high-angle environment, a *fall zone* is defined as the area:

    A. where you may safely free-fall.

    B. where you are most likely to encounter falling objects.

    C. immediately below the rescuer where it is safe to discard unnecessary equipment.

    D. that contains the most direct route to lower a patient on a backboard.

2. What are the four most common hazards associated with fire?

    A. Smoke, oxygen deficiency, high ambient temperatures, and toxic gases

    B. Oxygen deficiency, high ambient temperatures, toxic gases, and electric shock

    C. Smoke, oxygen deficiency, inhalation of tar particles, and injury from breaking glass

    D. High ambient temperatures, toxic gases, electric shock, and inhalation of tar particles

3. When trying to manage a disruptive patient, you should:

    A. turn your back on the patient to show him you are not a threat.

    B. attempt to disarm the patient yourself if he has a gun or knife.

    C. leave the patient alone for a few minutes to think about the situation.

    D. keep your eyes on the patient at all times and be alert for aggressive behavior.

4. Safety measures at the scene of an accident where there is a lot of glass and sharp metal objects should include wearing:

    A. cool, lightweight clothing to prevent sweating.

    B. sturdy work boots, leather gloves, and a hard hat.

    C. heavy rubberized boots, an overcoat, and a fire fighter's helmet.

    D. lightweight gloves so the hands are able to grip things easily.

Chapter 3

5. The appropriate course of action for handling a downed power line is to:

    A. push the line away with a long wooden pole.

    B. move the line while wearing electrician's gloves.

    C. establish a danger zone around the line without touching it.

    D. extinguish sparks and fire with an approved fire extinguisher.

6. To protect yourself from exposure to blood or other bodily fluids while in the field, you must wear:

    A. an oxygen mask.

    B. gloves, eye protection, and protective clothing.

    C. three layers of protective clothing.

    D. full turnout gear and an SCBA.

7. What gas attaches itself to the hemoglobin in red blood cells about 200 times more rapidly than oxygen, blocking the ability of the hemoglobin to transport oxygen to the body tissues?

    A. Carbon monoxide

    B. Carbon dioxide

    C. Hydrogen chloride

    D. Hydrogen cyanide

8. Water will draw body heat away how many times faster than air of the same temperature?

    A. 50

    B. 25

    C. 12

    D. 10

Personal Safety

9. A person with hypoxia may become excited, agitated, or confused as a result of low:

    A. blood pressure.

    B. oxygen levels.

    C. nitrogen levels.

    D. carbon dioxide levels.

10. What word is used in a fall zone to warn others of hard falling objects?

    A. Rope

    B. Rock

    C. Falling

    D. Hard

11. For traction on ice, mud, stainless steel chemical tanks, mold- or moss-covered rocks, or other hard surfaces that have a slippery covering, you should use:

    A. heavy, cleated hiking boots.

    B. structural firefighting boots.

    C. heavy-duty crampons.

    D. chest high waders.

12. Approximately what percent of room air is made up of oxygen?

    A. 25%

    B. 21%

    C. 19%

    D. 18%

13. When flying objects at a rescue scene are a possibility, you should:

    A. cease any rescue attempts.

    B. avoid using power extrication equipment.

    C. proceed as usual, as there is nothing you can do about them.

    D. take similar protective measures as those recommended for falling objects.

Chapter 3

14. In grain bins and silos, where the atmosphere may be highly saturated with grain dust, you must be particularly concerned because grain dust can:

    A. cause coughing, disabling the rescuers.

    B. consume a tremendous amount of oxygen.

    C. explode when exposed to a single spark.

    D. create carbon monoxide when in a confined space.

15. Tear gas destroys:

    A. lung tissue.

    B. skin layers.

    C. tear ducts.

    D. clothing.

16. Which of the following statements best defines a *backdraft*?

    A. It is the current formed when water rushes over a dam or natural obstacles in a river.

    B. It is the sudden ignition of all of the combustible items within a fire zone.

    C. It is a system of fans set up by the fire department to keep smoke out of the building.

    D. It is the explosion of gases emitted in the smoldering phase of the fire as the gases are mixed with additional oxygen.

17. What type of ventilation, when done properly, will allow the heated gases from a smoldering fire to escape a burning building in a controlled manner?

    A. Horizontal

    B. Vertical

    C. Angular

    D. Circular

16 Student Review Manual

Personal Safety

18. In snow or white sand, rescuers' eyes need protection from:

    A. the wind.

    B. whiteouts.

    C. excessive drying.

    D. ultraviolet radiation.

19. Which of the following is a colorless gas that has a strong, pungent odor and causes severe irritation to the respiratory tract and eyes?

    A. Phosgene

    B. Hydrogen chloride

    C. Carbon monoxide

    D. Carbon dioxide

20. Which of the following is a colorless gas that has the odor of musty hay and, in small amounts, can cause eye and throat irritation?

    A. Phosgene

    B. Hydrogen chloride

    C. Carbon monoxide

    D. Carbon dioxide

21. You are at the scene of a one-car accident in which a lone driver crashed into a tree. There is spilled gasoline around the automobile, and you see that the patient is unconscious, lying with his head leaning to the left near the window. As you approach the scene, your first step should be to:

    A. give the patient supplemental oxygen.

    B. pull the patient from the car immediately.

    C. call the fire department to wash down the scene.

    D. call a hazardous materials team to decontaminate the patient.

Chapter 3

22. What gas is responsible for more fire deaths each year than any other by-product of combustion?

    A. Hydrogen chloride

    B. Hydrogen cyanide

    C. Carbon dioxide

    D. Carbon monoxide

23. Prolonged exposure to cold may result in a potentially dangerous lowering of the body's core temperature known as:

    A. hyperthermia.

    B. hypothermia.

    C. hypertension.

    D. hypotension.

24. Prolonged exposure to heat that causes the internal body temperature to increase above normal is known as:

    A. hyperthermia.

    B. hypothermia.

    C. hypertension.

    D. hypotension.

25. Tissue damage resulting from exposure to low temperatures is called:

    A. hypothermia.

    B. hyperthermia.

    C. frostbite.

    D. trench foot.

Personal Safety

Answers

1: **B.** A *fall zone* is the area in a high-angle environment where you are most likely to encounter falling objects. (ECTSI 5, p. 43)

2: **A.** The four hazards commonly associated with fire are smoke, oxygen deficiency, high ambient temperatures, and toxic gases. (ECTSI 5, p. 35)

3: **D.** When trying to manage a disruptive patient, you should keep your eyes on the patient at all times and be alert for aggressive behavior. (ECTSI 5, p. 652)

4: **B.** Sturdy work boots, leather gloves, and a hard hat should be worn at an accident scene where there may be a lot of glass and sharp metal objects. (ECTSI 5, p. 704)

5: **C.** The appropriate course of action for handling a downed power line is to establish a danger zone around the line without touching it. You should not attempt to move downed power lines. You may use downed utility poles as landmarks for the perimeter of the danger zone, and then restrict the danger zone from entry by unauthorized personnel. (ECTSI 5, p. 41)

6: **B.** To protect yourself from exposure to blood or other bodily fluids while in the field, you should wear gloves, eye protection, and protective clothing. These are part of the universal precautions you should follow whenever exposure to blood or other bodily fluids is possible. (ECTSI 5, p. 30)

7: **A.** Carbon monoxide attaches itself to the hemoglobin in red blood cells about 200 times more rapidly than oxygen does, blocking the ability of the hemoglobin to transport oxygen to the body tissues. (ECTSI 5, p. 35)

8: **B.** Water draws body heat away 25 times faster than air of the same temperature. This is why there is a risk of rapidly developing hypothermia in cold water. (ECTSI 5, p. 39)

9: **B.** A person affected by hypoxia may become excited, agitated, or confused as a result of low oxygen levels. (ECTSI 5, p. 45)

10: **B.** The standard word used in a fall zone to warn others of a hard object falling is *rock*. (ECTSI 5, p. 43)

11: **C.** For traction on any slippery surface, it is best to use heavy-duty crampons, which are spiked metal plates that attach to boots or shoes. (ECTSI 5, p. 42)

Chapter 3

12: **B.** Approximately 21% of room air is made up of oxygen. (ECTSI 5, p. 45)

13: **D.** When power extrication tools are being used in a rescue situation, flying objects become a hazard. When flying objects are a possibility, similar protective measures as those recommended for falling objects should be taken. These include assuming a position that will allow your helmet to protect you and making your body as small a target as possible. (ECTSI 5, p. 44)

14: **C.** The atmosphere in grain bins may be highly saturated with grain dust, creating the potential for an explosion if the dust is exposed to even a single spark. (ECTSI 5, p. 45)

15: **A.** Lung tissue is destroyed by exposure to tear gas. (ECTSI 5, p. 46)

16: **D.** A backdraft occurs when gases are mixed with additional oxygen in the smoldering phase of a fire, causing them to explode. (ECTSI 5, p. 36)

17: **B.** Vertical ventilation, when done properly, will allow heated gases from a smoldering fire to escape a burning building in a controlled manner. (ECTSI 5, p. 37)

18: **D.** Special glasses or goggles are needed to protect rescuers' eyes from exposure to ultraviolet radiation that occurs when working in snow or white sand. (ECTSI 5, p. 34)

19: **B.** Hydrogen chloride is a colorless gas with a strong, pungent odor that causes severe irritation to the respiratory tract and eyes, and it may also result in an irregular heart beat. (ECTSI 5, p. 35)

20: **A.** Phosgene is a colorless gas with an odor of musty hay. Limited exposure to phosgene may result in eye and throat irritation. (ECTSI 5, p. 35)

21: **C.** The first step in this situation is to ensure the safety of both the rescue team and the patient. Therefore, your first step should be to call the fire department to wash down the scene. If gasoline or other flammable material is present, a fire crew with charged hoses should be standing by during the extrication process. (ECTSI 5, p. 705)

22: **D.** Carbon monoxide, which is present in every fire, is responsible for more fire deaths each year than any other by-product of combustion. (ECTSI 5, p. 35)

Personal Safety

23: **B.** Hypothermia, a potentially dangerous lowering of the body's core temperature, may develop after prolonged exposure to freezing or near-freezing temperatures. (ECTSI 5, p. 32)

24: **A.** Hyperthermia, the raising of the internal body temperature above normal, may develop after prolonged exposure to heat. (ECTSI 5, p. 32)

25: **C.** Tissue damage as a result of exposure to low temperatures is called frostbite. (ECTSI 5, p. 28)

Chapter 4

Basic Anatomy

Chapter Goals

The exercises in this chapter are designed to help the student to:

- define and use standard anatomic terms.

- identify the major topographic features of the body.

- describe the relationship between the external body landmarks and internal structures and organs.

Basic Anatomy

Multiple-Choice Questions

Select the correct answer for each of the following questions. Each question has only *one* correct or best answer.

1. Anatomically, the term *superior* means located:

    A. above.

    B. in front.

    C. in back.

    D. below.

2. The term *thorax* refers to the:

    A. brain case.

    B. back of the neck.

    C. pelvic cavity.

    D. chest.

3. The term *anterior* refers to the:

    A. front surface of the body.

    B. rear surface of the body.

    C. surface toward the midline.

    D. surface away from the midline.

4. The anatomic term for the *Adam's apple* is the:

    A. pharynx.

    B. larynx.

    C. esophagus.

    D. epiglottis.

Chapter 4

5. The superior boundary of the abdomen is the:

    A. diaphragm.

    B. pelvic girdle.

    C. posterior wall.

    D. anterior wall.

6. The *medial aspect* of a bone is that part of a bone:

    A. toward the midline.

    B. away from the midline.

    C. nearer to the back.

    D. nearer a free end.

7. The inferior boundary of the thorax is the:

    A. diaphragm.

    B. pelvic girdle.

    C. midline.

    D. abdomen.

8. Anatomically, the term *distal* means located:

    A. nearer the trunk.

    B. on the front surface.

    C. toward the midline.

    D. away from the midline.

9. The largest single organ of the body is the:

    A. heart.

    B. brain.

    C. liver.

    D. skin.

Basic Anatomy

10. The *inferior aspect* of an organ is that part of the organ:

    A. toward the head.

    B. toward the feet.

    C. toward the midline.

    D. away from the midline.

11. The bone that forms the lower jaw is the:

    A. mastoid.

    B. maxilla.

    C. mandible.

    D. cranium.

12. In the neck, the esophagus lies:

    A. anterior to the trachea.

    B. posterior to the cervical vertebrae.

    C. posterior to the trachea.

    D. within the cricoid cartilage.

13. The flap of tissue that acts to prevent food or liquid from entering the lungs is called the:

    A. trachea.

    B. bronchus.

    C. epiglottis.

    D. larynx.

14. The shoulder girdle is composed of what three bones?

    A. Clavicle, scapula, femur

    B. Clavicle, scapula, humerus

    C. Sternum, clavicle, humerus

    D. Sternum, clavicle, femur

Chapter 4

15. The three major structures of the thorax are the:

    A. esophagus, trachea, and larynx.

    B. heart, lungs, and spleen.

    C. heart, lungs, and esophagus.

    D. stomach, lungs, and liver.

16. Which of the following bones is found in the foot?

    A. Acromion

    B. Calcaneus

    C. Patella

    D. Olecranon

17. The heart lies in the chest:

    A. superior to the lungs.

    B. at the level of the seventh to the tenth ribs.

    C. completely to the right of the midline.

    D. immediately posterior to the sternum.

18. Most of the stomach lies in what quadrant of the abdomen?

    A. Left upper

    B. Left lower

    C. Right lower

    D. Right upper

19. The pelvis is composed of the sacrum and the innominate bone. The innominate bone is a fusion of the:

    A. femur and the pubis.

    B. lumbar vertebrae.

    C. ilium, the ischium, and the pubis.

    D. greater and lesser trochanters.

Basic Anatomy

20. What major artery supplies blood to the lower extremity?

    A. Carotid

    B. Femoral

    C. Subclavian

    D. Brachial

21. The head is divided into what two parts?

    A. Cranium and face

    B. Cranium and occiput

    C. Temporal and parietal regions

    D. Frontal region and the base

22. The cartilaginous tip of the sternum is called the:

    A. manubrium.

    B. xiphoid process.

    C. angle of Louis.

    D. jugular notch.

23. The longest, strongest bone in the body is the:

    A. tibia.

    B. femur.

    C. fibula.

    D. humerus.

24. Eight carpal bones form the basis of the:

    A. knee.

    B. wrist.

    C. cervical spine.

    D. lumbar spine.

Chapter 4

25. Of the following, which is considered one of the great vessels?

   A. Carotid artery

   B. Jugular vein

   C. Femoral artery

   D. Inferior vena cava

Answers

1: **A.** The term *superior* refers to a point or structure above another (e.g., the humerus is superior to the radius and ulna.) (ECTSI 5, p. 52)

2: **D.** The thorax is the chest area. (ECTSI 5, p. 55)

3: **A.** The term *anterior* refers to the front surface of the body. (ECTSI 5, p. 52)

4: **B.** The larynx may protrude from the anterior surface of the neck. It is known as the *Adam's apple*. (ECTSI 5, p. 54)

5: **A.** The diaphragm is the superior boundary of the abdomen. (ECTSI 5, pp. 56–57)

6: **A.** The term *medial* means toward the midline of the body. (ECTSI 5, p. 52)

7: **A.** The inferior boundary of the thorax is the diaphragm. The diaphragm separates the thorax from the abdomen. (ECTSI 5, p. 56)

8: **D.** *Distal* refers to a point farther away from the midline of the body, or some other reference point. Proximal refers to a nearer point. (ECTSI 5, p. 52)

9: **D.** The single largest organ of the body is the skin. (ECTSI 5, p. 231)

10: **B.** The term *inferior* refers to a position toward the feet, or to an organ or structure lying below another. (ECTSI 5, p. 52)

11: **C.** The mandible forms the lower jaw. (ECTSI 5, p. 53)

12: **C.** The esophagus lies posterior to, or behind, the trachea. (ECTSI 5, p. 102)

13: **C.** The epiglottis closes over the opening to the trachea whenever food or liquid is present in the pharynx. (ECTSI 5, p. 103)

Basic Anatomy

14: **B.** The shoulder girdle is composed of the clavicle anteriorly, the scapula posteriorly, and the upper end of the humerus laterally. (ECTSI 5, p. 61)

15: **C.** The heart, lungs, and esophagus are the three major structures located in the thorax. (ECTSI 5, p. 55)

16: **B.** The bones in the foot include the malleoli in the ankle, and the talus, calcaneus, metatarsals, and phalanges. (ECTSI 5, pp. 60–61)

17: **D.** The heart lies immediately posterior to, or underneath, the sternum. (ECTSI 5, p. 56)

18: **A.** Most of the stomach lies in the left upper quadrant of the abdomen, protected by the lower portion of the left rib cage. (ECTSI 5, p. 57)

19: **C.** The innominate bone is a fusion of the ilium, ischium, and pubis. It connects with the sacrum to form the ring of bone called the pelvis. (ECTSI 5, p. 59)

20: **B.** The femoral artery supplies blood to the lower extremity. (ECTSI 5, pp. 63, 138)

21: **A.** The head is divided into two parts: the cranium and the face. (ECTSI 5, p. 53)

22: **B.** The sternum has three components: the manubrium, the body, and the xiphoid process. The upper quarter of the sternum is the manubrium. The body comprises the rest, except for the narrow cartilaginous tip inferiorly, called the xiphoid process. (ECTSI 5, p. 55)

23: **B.** The femur is the supporting bone of the thigh and is considered the longest, strongest bone in the body. (ECTSI 5, p. 60)

24: **B.** There are eight bones, called carpal bones, in the wrist. (ECTSI 5, p. 62)

25: **D.** The great vessels are those entering or leaving the heart, including the aorta, the pulmonary arteries and veins, and the venae cavae. (ECTSI 5, pp. 56–57, 137)

Chapter 5

Assessing Vital Signs

Chapter Goals

The exercises in this chapter are designed to help the student to:

- distinguish between signs and symptoms.

- identify the normal range of vital signs for adults, children, and infants.

- describe the importance of mechanism of injury and patient history in providing appropriate emergency care.

- identify the sequence of assessment and treatment priorities.

Assessing Vital Signs

Multiple-Choice Questions

Select the correct answer for each of the following questions. Each question has only *one* correct or best answer.

1. The normal heart rate of an average, healthy adult is approximately how many beats per minute?

    A. 12 to 16

    B. 20 to 40

    C. 60 to 100

    D. 100 plus the adult's age

2. The normal respiratory rate of an average, healthy adult is approximately how many breaths per minute?

    A. 6 to 12

    B. 12 to 20

    C. 20 to 25

    D. 26 to 30

3. Pulse volume, often described as regular, thready, or bounding, is a general indication of the:

    A. heart's rhythm.

    B. strength of the heart's contractions.

    C. amount of blockage in the arteries.

    D. temperature of the blood.

4. The best way to evaluate the radial pulse is to use the:

    A. palm of your hand.

    B. thumb.

    C. back of your hand.

    D. tips of your fingers.

Chapter 5

5. Pulse is defined as the:

    A. pressure wave of blood that is felt as the heart sends blood through an artery.

    B. swelling of a vein as each pressure wave of blood passes back to the heart.

    C. number of heart beats in the column of blood in a large vein.

    D. vibration of the heart muscles as they push blood through the blood vessels.

6. Cyanosis may be seen in patients with deeply pigmented skin by observing the:

    A. knuckles.

    B. abdomen.

    C. nail beds.

    D. ear lobes.

7. Evaluating pupillary reaction is important during assessment to monitor changes in:

    A. neurologic status.

    B. blood pressure.

    C. retinal pressure.

    D. circulation.

8. An adult male patient has what is considered to be a serious condition if his baseline systolic blood pressure is below:

    A. 150 mm Hg.

    B. 125 mm Hg.

    C. 100 mm Hg.

    D. 90 mm Hg.

Assessing Vital Signs

9. The appropriate way to assess a systolic blood pressure by auscultation is to:

   A. note the point on the gauge at which the sound disappears or changes in quality.

   B. note the point on the gauge at which the needle starts moving.

   C. note the point on the gauge at which you first hear a strong sound.

   D. inflate the bulb of the blood pressure cuff until it reaches 200 mm Hg.

10. The radial pulse is palpated:

    A. in the groin.

    B. at the inner aspect of the elbow.

    C. at the wrist proximal to the thumb.

    D. in the neck below the angle of the jaw.

11. A bounding pulse feels:

    A. normal.

    B. stronger than normal.

    C. weaker than normal.

    D. barely palpable.

12. A sign differs from a symptom in that a sign is:

    A. observed by the EMT.

    B. reported by the patient.

    C. reported by the physician.

    D. recorded in the medical record, whereas a symptom is not.

13. A pulse is most readily felt at points where the artery is:

    A. close to the skin.

    B. close to cartilage.

    C. located directly over a bone.

    D. located both close to the skin and directly over a bone.

Chapter 5

14. The normal heart rate for an average, healthy 10-year-old child is approximately how many beats per minute?

    A. 16 to 20

    B. 30 to 50

    C. 80 to 100

    D. 100 plus the child's age

15. Normal systolic blood pressure in an adult male is approximately:

    A. 90 mm Hg plus the patient's age, not to exceed 150 mm Hg.

    B. 95 mm Hg plus the patient's age, not to exceed 150 mm Hg.

    C. 100 mm Hg plus the patient's age, not to exceed 150 mm Hg.

    D. 105 mm Hg plus the patient's age, not to exceed 150 mm Hg.

16. You should take a patient's carotid pulse if the:

    A. radial pulse is bounding.

    B. radial pulse cannot be palpated.

    C. patient has a head injury.

    D. patient has traumatic chest injuries.

17. When evaluating respirations, you should observe and record:

    A. rate and rhythm.

    B. rate and degree of chest movement.

    C. rhythm and degree of chest movement.

    D. rate and character of respirations.

Assessing Vital Signs

18. Normal systolic blood pressure in an adult female is approximately:

    A. 65 to 90 mm Hg.

    B. 100 mm Hg plus the patient's age.

    C. 8 to 10 mm Hg lower than that of a male of the same age and physical condition.

    D. 10 to 20 mm Hg higher than that of a male of the same age and physical condition.

19. After you assess a patient's blood pressure, you should record the values, the extremity in which the pressure was taken, and the:

    A. position of the patient.

    B. type of blood pressure cuff.

    C. location of the stethoscope.

    D. type of injury or suspected condition.

20. Labored or difficult breathing is called:

    A. apnea.

    B. dyspnea.

    C. hyperpnea.

    D. orthopnea.

21. The blood pressure cuff should be wrapped snugly around the upper extremity, with the lower edge of the cuff:

    A. 1 inch above the elbow.

    B. 1 inch below the armpit.

    C. 2 inches above the elbow.

    D. 2 inches below the armpit.

Chapter 5

22. The heart rate of an average, healthy newborn is typically how many beats per minute?

    A. 40 to 60

    B. 60 to 100

    C. 120 to 140

    D. 160 to 200

23. You are taking a blood pressure by palpation. As the cuff is deflated, you should note and record the value on the gauge when the:

    A. needle begins to move.

    B. pulse sounds first appear.

    C. pulse sounds disappear.

    D. radial pulse is felt.

24. The pulse rate of an average, healthy adult is typically between:

    A. 15 and 40 per minute.

    B. 40 and 60 per minute.

    C. 60 and 100 per minute.

    D. 100 plus the adult's age per minute.

25. Assessment of the circulatory system includes evaluating a patient's:

    A. pupillary reactions.

    B. capillary refill.

    C. level of consciousness.

    D. response to pain.

Assessing Vital Signs

Answers

1: **C.** The normal heart rate of an average, healthy adult is approximately 60 to 100 beats per minute. (ECTSI 5, p. 67)

2: **B.** The normal respiratory rate of an average, healthy adult is approximately 12 to 20 breaths per minute. (ECTSI 5, p. 68)

3: **B.** Pulse volume is considered a rough indicator of the strength of the heart's contractions. (ECTSI 5, p. 68)

4: **D.** The best way to evaluate the radial pulse is to use the tips of your fingers. (ECTSI 5, pp. 80–81)

5: **A.** The pulse is the pressure wave or surge of blood moving through an artery as a result of contractions of the heart. (ECTSI 5, p. 66)

6: **C.** The nail beds of deeply pigmented people will show a bluish tint if cyanosis is present. The mucous membranes inside the mouth and the sclera ("white") of the eye will also show cyanosis. (ECTSI 5, p. 72)

7: **A.** Assessing pupillary reaction is important for monitoring changes in neurologic status. (ECTSI 5, p. 75)

8: **D.** While normal baseline systolic blood pressure will vary from patient to patient, a reading of 90 mm Hg indicates a serious condition, particularly if it is a lower value than that found in a previous reading. (ECTSI 5, pp. 71, 212)

9: **C.** The point at which you first hear the sound of a pulse wave is the patient's systolic blood pressure. The diastolic blood pressure is noted when the sound disappears. (ECTSI 5, pp. 70–71)

10: **C.** The radial pulse is palpated at the wrist, proximal to the thumb. (ECTSI 5, p. 67)

11: **B.** A bounding pulse feels stronger than normal. (ECTSI 5, p. 68)

12: **A.** A sign is something that you observe in a patient, such as a deformity, bleeding, or a patient's blood pressure. (ECTSI 5, p. 66)

13: **D.** A pulse is most readily palpated where the artery is located both close to the skin and over a bone. (ECTSI 5, p. 66)

Chapter 5

14: **C.** The normal heart rate for an average, healthy child is approximately 80 to 100 beats per minute. (ECTSI 5, p. 67)

15: **C.** Normal systolic blood pressure in an adult male is 100 mm Hg plus the patient's age, not to exceed 150 mm Hg. (ECTSI 5, p. 71)

16: **B.** The carotid pulse should be taken if the radial pulse cannot be palpated. (ECTSI 5, p. 67)

17: **D.** Rate and character of respirations, including chest movement, should be assessed when evaluating respirations. (ECTSI 5, p. 68)

18: **C.** Blood pressure in an average adult female is 8 to 10 mm Hg lower than that of a comparable male. (ECTSI 5, p. 71)

19: **A.** The record of a blood pressure measurement should include the values, the extremity in which the pressure was taken, and the position of the patient. (ECTSI 5, p. 71)

20: **B.** Dyspnea describes air hunger resulting in difficult or labored breathing. (ECTSI 5, p. 467)

21: **A.** The correct placement of the blood pressure cuff is 1" above the elbow. (ECTSI 5, p. 70)

22: **C.** The heart rate of an average, healthy newborn is typically between 120 and 140 beats per minute. (ECTSI 5, pp. 67–68)

23: **D.** When taking the blood pressure by palpation, the point at which the radial pulse is felt indicates the value. (ECTSI 5, p. 70)

24: **C.** The normal pulse rate of an average, healthy adult is between 60 and 100 beats per minute. (ECTSI 5, p. 67)

25: **B.** Assessment of the circulatory system includes evaluating capillary refill, pulse rate, skin temperature, skin color, and skin moisture. (ECTSI 5, pp. 80–81)

Chapter 6

The Respiratory and Circulatory Systems

Chapter Goals

The exercises in this chapter are designed to help the student to:

- identify the parts of the respiratory system.

- identify the parts of the circulatory system.

- describe the breathing process.

- describe how blood circulates in the body.

- explain how the respiratory and circulatory systems work together to bring oxygen to the cells and expel carbon dioxide.

Chapter 6

Multiple-Choice Questions

Select the correct answer for each of the following questions. Each question has only *one* correct or best answer.

1. The phase of breathing that occurs when the chest muscles contract and the lungs expand and fill with air is called:

    A. respiration.

    B. expiration.

    C. inspiration.

    D. ventilation.

2. The flap of tissue that allows air to enter the lungs, but prevents food or liquid to enter, is called the:

    A. trachea.

    B. bronchus.

    C. epiglottis.

    D. larynx.

3. Of the two tubes that extend downward from the throat, the one that carries air to the lungs is called the:

    A. trachea.

    B. bronchus.

    C. pharynx.

    D. esophagus.

4. Oxygen and carbon dioxide are exchanged in the lungs through the walls of the pulmonary:

    A. arteries.

    B. veins.

    C. capillaries.

    D. venules.

The Respiratory and Circulatory Systems

5. The volume of air that moves through the alveoli every 60 seconds is called the:

    A. residual volume.

    B. minute volume.

    C. tidal volume.

    D. reserve volume.

6. Of the two tubes that extend downward from the throat, the one that carries ingested food to the stomach is called the:

    A. trachea.

    B. esophagus.

    C. larynx.

    D. epiglottis.

7. Deoxygenated blood is carried to the lungs from the:

    A. left ventricle.

    B. left atrium.

    C. right ventricle.

    D. right atrium.

8. Oxygenated blood is carried away from the heart through the aorta into the:

    A. arteries.

    B. veins.

    C. capillaries.

    D. venules.

9. The air we inhale contains about how much oxygen?

    A. 16%

    B. 21%

    C. 40%

    D. 80%

Chapter 6

10. The air we exhale contains about how much oxygen?

    A. 16%

    B. 21%

    C. 40%

    D. 80%

11. The rate and depth of breathing are regulated by the:

    A. brain.

    B. diaphragm.

    C. intercostal muscles.

    D. spinal cord.

12. Expiration occurs when the intercostal muscles and the diaphragm:

    A. contract.

    B. expand.

    C. relax.

    D. tense.

13. When you inhale, the intercostal muscles and the diaphragm:

    A. contract.

    B. expand.

    C. relax.

    D. tense.

14. The backup system for controlling respiration is called:

    A. diffusion.

    B. the hypoxic drive.

    C. metabolism.

    D. carbon dioxide exchange.

The Respiratory and Circulatory Systems

15. Breathing is usually controlled by the brain's sensitivity to the blood's level of:

    A. oxygen.

    B. carbon dioxide.

    C. carbon monoxide.

    D. nitrogen.

16. Which of the following is the largest artery that carries freshly oxygenated blood to the body?

    A. Radial

    B. Femoral

    C. Aorta

    D. Brachial

17. The lungs are each covered by a smooth, glistening, membranous sac called the:

    A. visceral pleura.

    B. parietal pleura.

    C. diaphragm.

    D. mesentery.

18. The diaphragm is considered a unique muscle in that it has:

    A. both voluntary and involuntary functions.

    B. striated markings.

    C. the capability to both contract and relax at the same time.

    D. a thin film of fluid that lubricates the rib cage.

19. Blood is carried to the heart by the:

    A. arteries.

    B. veins.

    C. capillaries.

    D. arterioles.

Chapter 6

20. The function of the pulmonary circulation is to carry:

    A. oxygenated blood through the body and deoxygenated blood to the heart.

    B. deoxygenated blood through the lungs and oxygenated blood to the heart.

    C. oxygenated blood through the lungs and deoxygenated blood to the heart.

    D. deoxygenated blood through the body and oxygenated blood to the heart.

21. The function of the systemic circulation is to carry:

    A. oxygenated blood through the body and deoxygenated blood to the heart.

    B. deoxygenated blood through the lungs and oxygenated blood to the heart.

    C. oxygenated blood through the lungs and deoxygenated blood to the heart.

    D. deoxygenated blood through the body and oxygenated blood to the heart.

22. The average adult male body contains about how many pints of blood?

    A. 8

    B. 10

    C. 12

    D. 15

23. The solid components of blood needed for gas transport in respiration are contained in the:

    A. erythrocytes.

    B. leukocytes.

    C. platelets.

    D. plasma.

24. The solid components of blood needed for clotting are contained in the:

    A. erythrocytes.

    B. leukocytes.

    C. platelets.

    D. plasma.

The Respiratory and Circulatory Systems

25. The solid components of blood that help the body protect itself against infection are contained in the:

    A. erythrocytes.

    B. leukocytes.

    C. platelets.

    D. plasma.

26. The brachial artery supplies blood to the:

    A. brain.

    B. upper extremity.

    C. lower extremity.

    D. myocardium.

27. The fluid component of blood is found in the:

    A. erythrocytes.

    B. leukocytes.

    C. platelets.

    D. plasma.

28. The exchange of oxygen for carbon dioxide and other cellular waste materials takes place in the walls of the:

    A. arteries.

    B. veins.

    C. capillaries.

    D. arterioles.

29. Arteries can constrict or dilate because their walls are lined with a layer of:

    A. elastic tissue.

    B. striated muscle.

    C. smooth muscle.

    D. voluntary muscle.

Chapter 6

30. The structures in veins that prevent the backward flow of blood are called:

   A. valves.

   B. fibrils.

   C. tendrils.

   D. glands.

Answers

1: **C.** Inspiration is the phase of breathing where the lungs expand and fill with air. (ECTSI 5, p. 105)

2: **C.** The epiglottis is a thin, leaf-shaped flap of tissue that allows only air to enter the trachea. (ECTSI 5, p. 103)

3: **A.** The trachea carries air to the lungs. It is in front of the esophagus, which carries food and liquid into the stomach. (ECTSI 5, p. 102)

4: **C.** Oxygen and carbon dioxide are exchanged in the lungs through the pulmonary capillaries. (ECTSI 5, p. 102)

5: **B.** Minute volume is the amount of air that moves through the alveoli every 60 seconds. (ECTSI 5, p. 173)

6: **B.** The esophagus carries ingested food from the pharynx into the stomach. (ECTSI 5, pp. 102–103)

7. **C.** Deoxygenated blood is carried from the right ventricle through the lungs and back to the left atrium. (ECTSI 5, p. 133)

8: **A.** Oxygenated blood is carried away from the heart through the aorta into the arteries. Arteries gradually become smaller (arterioles); here the blood finally passes into the capillaries. (ECTSI 5, pp. 133–134)

9: **B.** Inhaled air contains 21% oxygen and 78% nitrogen. Small amounts of other gases make up the final 1%. (ECTSI 5, p. 101)

10: **A.** Exhaled air contains 16% oxygen and 3% to 5% carbon dioxide. The remainder consists of nitrogen. (ECTSI 5, p. 102)

11: **A.** The brain controls the rate and depth of breathing. The center for this control is in the brainstem, which monitors the level of carbon dioxide in the blood. (ECTSI 5, p. 106)

The Respiratory and Circulatory Systems

12: **C.** The intercostal muscles and diaphragm relax, the chest cavity becomes smaller, and air moves from the lungs during expiration. (ECTSI 5, pp. 105–106)

13: **A.** Inhalation is the active muscular part of breathing in which the intercostal muscles and diaphragm contract. (ECTSI 5, p. 105)

14: **B.** The hypoxic drive is the backup system that controls respiration. (ECTSI 5, p. 106)

15: **B.** The level of carbon dioxide in the blood controls breathing. (ECTSI 5, p. 106)

16: **C.** The aorta is the major vessel leaving the left side of the heart carrying oxygenated blood to the body. (ECTSI 5, p. 136)

17: **A.** The lungs are each covered by visceral pleura, which is made up of smooth, glistening, membranous tissue. (ECTSI 5, p. 104)

18: **A.** The diaphragm is unique in that it has both voluntary and involuntary functions. (ECTSI 5, p. 105)

19: **B.** Blood returns to the right atrium of the heart through the veins. (ECTSI 5, p. 137)

20: **B.** Pulmonary circulation carries deoxygenated blood through the lungs where it is then oxygenated and carried to the heart. (ECTSI 5, p. 133)

21: **A.** Systemic circulation carries oxygenated blood from the heart, through the body and deoxygenated blood to the heart. (ECTSI 5, p. 133)

22: **C.** The normal blood volume in an average adult male is 12 pints, or about 6 liters. (ECTSI 5, p. 140)

23: **A.** Erythrocytes (red blood cells) are needed for gas transport during respiration. (ECTSI 5, p. 135)

24: **C.** Platelets are needed for the initial formation of blood clots. (ECTSI 5, p. 135)

25: **B.** Leukocytes (white blood cells) help to protect the body against infection. (ECTSI 5, p. 135)

26: **B.** The brachial arteries and their branches carry oxygenated blood to the upper extremities. (ECTSI 5, p. 138)

American Academy of Orthopaedic Surgeons

Chapter 6

27: **D.** Plasma is the sticky, yellow fluid component of blood that carries blood cells and nutrients. (ECTSI 5, p. 135)

28: **C.** The exchange of oxygen for carbon dioxide and other cellular waste materials takes place in the capillaries. (ECTSI 5, p. 134)

29: **C.** Arterial walls contain a layer of smooth muscle tissue. (ECTSI 5, p. 134)

30: **A.** Valves within the veins prevent the backward flow of blood. (ECTSI 5, p. 135)

Chapter 7

Cardiopulmonary Resuscitation and Basic Life Support

Chapter Goals

The exercises in this chapter are designed to help the student to:

- describe the effects of cardiac arrest on the body.

- define BLS and its urgency during cardiac arrest.

- describe the EMT's responsibilities for starting and stopping CPR.

- identify the four techniques for opening the airway.

- describe the various techniques for artificial ventilation and their appropriate uses.

- describe the various techniques for artificial circulation and their appropriate uses.

- explain the differences in providing CPR for infants and children, when compared with adults.

- identify the signs and symptoms of foreign body airway obstruction in adults, children, and infants.

- describe proper care of foreign body airway obstruction in adults, children, and infants.

Chapter 7

Multiple-Choice Questions

Select the correct answer for each of the following questions. Each question has only *one* correct or best answer.

1. Within seconds of being deprived of oxygen, the heart will develop:

    A. necrosis.

    B. scar tissue.

    C. arrhythmias.

    D. congestive heart failure.

2. Which of the following patients would **NOT** require immediate basic life support?

    A. A child in respiratory arrest

    B. A man with a complete airway obstruction

    C. An elderly woman with a fractured metatarsal

    D. A woman who has severe bleeding from a chest injury

3. A patient who is pulseless for more than 6 minutes is most likely to have:

    A. a stroke.

    B. brain damage.

    C. congestive heart failure.

    D. angina.

4. Early, effective basic life support measures are **NOT** likely to resuscitate a patient who has:

    A. been struck by lightning.

    B. been in ventricular fibrillation.

    C. had a foreign body obstruction.

    D. had a near-drowning accident.

Cardiopulmonary Resuscitation and Basic Life Support

5. A 65-year-old man has fallen off the roof and is lying facedown on the ground. He does not appear to be breathing, and you suspect that he may have a neck or back injury. The appropriate course of action is to:

   A. roll him into a supine position keeping his head, neck, and back aligned, assess his ABCs, and begin basic life support if necessary.

   B. place him in the recovery position, assess his ABCs, and begin basic life support if necessary.

   C. place him in a supine position by rolling him away from you, assess his ABCs, and begin basic life support if necessary.

   D. give him back blows to start him breathing, turn him over into a supine position, and give him mouth-to-mouth resuscitation.

6. Which of the following is considered a basic life support skill?

   A. Heimlich maneuver

   B. Cardiac monitoring

   C. Intravenous fluid therapy

   D. Medication administration

7. Patients with terminal illnesses often prepare legal documents that inform EMS providers that when they die, CPR should not be started. What are these documents called?

   A. Run reports

   B. Local protocols

   C. Nursing notes

   D. Living wills

8. Which of the following is **NOT** an acceptable reason for you to stop resuscitation once you have started?

   A. You are too fatigued and exhausted to continue any longer.

   B. The patient starts breathing on his own and you feel a pulse.

   C. A bystander tells you he thinks that the patient has a living will.

   D. A physician at the scene assumes responsibility and tells you to stop.

Chapter 7

9. You find your 70-year-old neighbor in full cardiac arrest on the front porch of her house. Another neighbor tells you that he does not think you should start CPR because he knows the woman was depressed and did not care about her life. You start CPR based on what legal principle?

    A. Implied consent

    B. Informed consent

    C. Good Samaritan laws

    D. Involuntary Treatment Act

10. A nontrauma patient should be transported in which of the following positions to facilitate spontaneous breathing and to allow for secretions to drain from the mouth?

    A. Supine position

    B. Recovery position

    C. Trendelenburg's position

    D. Resuscitation position

11. What is the most common cause of airway obstruction in an unconscious adult?

    A. Severe bleeding due to trauma

    B. Inhaling noxious or toxic materials

    C. Experiencing an anaphylactic reaction to a bee sting

    D. Relaxing of the muscles in the throat and tongue

12. What is the most commonly used method for opening the airway of a nontrauma patient?

    A. Sellick maneuver

    B. Head-tilt maneuver

    C. Neck-lift maneuver

    D. Heimlich maneuver

Cardiopulmonary Resuscitation and Basic Life Support

13. A patient suddenly slumps forward and stops breathing as you are taking his blood pressure. He still has a pulse. You should immediately start:

    A. artificial ventilation.

    B. external chest compressions.

    C. cardiopulmonary resuscitation.

    D. a blind finger sweep of the mouth.

14. CPR should be started if a patient has obvious signs of:

    A. lividity.

    B. rigor mortis.

    C. putrefaction.

    D. head injury with cardiac arrest.

15. You are alone at the scene of an accident in which you have determined that the patient is unresponsive and in need of CPR. Your first step in caring for the patient is to:

    A. start full CPR.

    B. activate the EMS system.

    C. administer high-flow oxygen.

    D. obtain a complete set of vital signs.

16. You are called to the home of a 40-year-old man in cardiac arrest. A neighbor says she thinks the patient signed a living will requesting no CPR, but she cannot produce the document. The most appropriate course of action would be to:

    A. immediately start CPR.

    B. wait for the neighbor to locate the living will.

    C. wait until you can contact medical control for instructions.

    D. transfer the patient to the ambulance, and then start BLS.

Chapter 7

17. For CPR to be effective, the patient must be placed on a firm surface in what position?

    A. Prone

    B. Vertical

    C. Supine

    D. Side-lying

18. Airway obstruction will often develop in an unconscious patient when there is relaxation of the:

    A. uvula.

    B. tongue.

    C. chest wall.

    D. diaphragm.

19. Which of the following is **LEAST** likely to cause airway obstruction?

    A. Vomitus

    B. Blood clots

    C. Loose dentures

    D. Nasal flaring

20. The jaw-thrust maneuver is best performed when you are positioned:

    A. kneeling above the patient's head.

    B. lying parallel to the patient's body.

    C. straddling across the patient's hips.

    D. squatting next to the patient's knees.

Cardiopulmonary Resuscitation and Basic Life Support

21. A patient with which of the following conditions will best tolerate the jaw-thrust maneuver?

    A. Moderate dyspnea

    B. Deep unconsciousness

    C. Mild bronchospasm

    D. Prolonged diarrhea

22. If untreated, a patient in respiratory arrest may die due to:

    A. ataxia.

    B. anoxia.

    C. hypocarbia.

    D. hypovolemia.

23. Adequate ventilations require inspirations that last for about how many seconds?

    A. 1/2 to 1

    B. 1 1/2 to 2

    C. 3 to 4

    D. 5 to 6

24. During mouth-to-mask ventilation, without the use of supplemental oxygen, exhaled air from the rescuer will contain what percentage of oxygen?

    A. 16%

    B. 21%

    C. 26%

    D. 35%

Chapter 7

25. Mouth-to-mask ventilation is effective if:

    A. the patient's chest rises and falls.

    B. air escapes during inhalation.

    C. the lungs fail to expand.

    D. the patient's pupils become equally dilated.

26. Which of the following ventilation techniques should be used for a patient who has had a laryngectomy?

    A. Mouth to mask

    B. Mouth to stoma

    C. Mouth to mouth

    D. Mouth to nose

27. What is one of the most common side effects of artificial ventilation?

    A. Acute epiglottitis

    B. Gastric distention

    C. Massive hemothorax

    D. Tension pneumothorax

28. Which of the following objects is **LEAST** likely to cause upper airway obstruction?

    A. Blood clots

    B. Bone fragments

    C. Ruptured alveoli

    D. Dislodged dentures

Cardiopulmonary Resuscitation and Basic Life Support

29. Gastric distention during artificial ventilation is considered dangerous because it can:

    A. stimulate hyperventilation.

    B. result in bacterial pneumonia.

    C. cause regurgitation and aspiration of stomach contents during CPR.

    D. increase total lung volume by elevating the diaphragm.

30. Sudden foreign body airway obstruction in adults usually occurs during:

    A. meals.

    B. nightmares.

    C. panic attacks.

    D. athletic activity.

31. Which of the following does **NOT** usually occur when a conscious adult has a sudden foreign body airway obstruction?

    A. Cyanosis

    B. Sudden chills

    C. Inability to speak

    D. Grasping at the throat

32. What are the two manual maneuvers recommended for relieving foreign body airway obstruction in adults?

    A. Precordial thumps and back blows

    B. Abdominal thrusts and back blows

    C. Abdominal thrusts and finger sweeps

    D. Finger sweeps and precordial thumps

Chapter 7

33. In most instances, cardiac arrest in infants and children results from:

    A. unwitnessed electrocution.

    B. severe head trauma.

    C. severe hypothermia.

    D. respiratory arrest.

34. What is the recommended technique for opening the airway of a child?

    A. Head-tilt/chin-lift maneuver

    B. Chin-lift maneuver

    C. Jaw-thrust/head-tilt maneuver

    D. Modified jaw-thrust maneuver

35. A newborn infant should be ventilated how many times a minute?

    A. 10

    B. 20

    C. 30

    D. 40

36. Of the following, which is **LEAST** likely to cause upper airway obstruction in an infant or child?

    A. Croup

    B. A foreign body

    C. Epiglottitis

    D. Pneumonia

37. What is the most common arrhythmia, occurring in up to 70% of all cardiac arrests?

    A. Atrial fibrillation

    B. Sinus tachycardia

    C. Junctional tachycardia

    D. Ventricular fibrillation

Cardiopulmonary Resuscitation and Basic Life Support

38. Which of the following is **NOT** a sign of poor air exchange in a child?

    A. Cyanosis

    B. Flushed skin

    C. Ineffective cough

    D. Stridorous breathing

39. Pulseless electrical activity (PEA) is a form of cardiac arrest in which the:

    A. heart has no electrical or detectable muscular activity.

    B. ventricles beat so fast there is not enough time for the pumping chambers to fill between beats.

    C. pumping chambers of the heart experience continuous chaotic, uncoordinated muscular quivering.

    D. cardiac monitor shows adequate heart rate and rhythm, but there is no detectable pulse or blood pressure.

40. Placing your hands over the xiphoid process when performing chest compressions on an adult can result in:

    A. fractured ribs.

    B. effective CPR.

    C. pulmonary embolus.

    D. laceration of the liver.

41. Currently, what is the appropriate ratio of compressions to relaxations during adult CPR?

    A. 60% compressions to 40% relaxations

    B. 50% compressions to 50% relaxations

    C. 30% compressions to 70% relaxations

    D. 40% compressions to 60% relaxations

Chapter 7

42. To monitor the effectiveness of single-rescuer adult CPR, the carotid pulse should be palpated for:

    A. 5 seconds after the first minute of CPR, and then every 5 minutes thereafter.

    B. 5 seconds after the first 5 minutes of CPR, and then every minute thereafter.

    C. 10 seconds after the first 2 minutes of CPR, and then every 2 minutes thereafter.

    D. 10 seconds after the first minute of CPR, and then every 3 minutes thereafter.

43. Except when it is absolutely necessary to move a patient, CPR should not be interrupted for more than how many seconds?

    A. 5

    B. 10

    C. 15

    D. 20

44. For a patient in cardiac arrest, basic life support measures alone will rarely be sufficient for survival without the addition of:

    A. defibrillation.

    B. nitroglycerin.

    C. supplemental oxygen.

    D. the Heimlich maneuver.

45. In infants, which pulse should be palpated to assess the quality of the pulse?

    A. Brachial

    B. Radial

    C. Carotid

    D. Popliteal

Cardiopulmonary Resuscitation and Basic Life Support

46. The proper way to perform chest compressions on an infant is with:

    A. two fingers placed at midsternum.

    B. two fingers placed on the lower sternum.

    C. the heel of one hand placed at midsternum.

    D. the heel of one hand placed on the lower sternum.

47. What is the proper chest compression rate for infants and children?

    A. 60/min

    B. 75/min

    C. 100/min

    D. 125/min

48. What is the proper ratio of compressions to ventilations for one-rescuer adult CPR?

    A. 1:5

    B. 2:15

    C. 5:1

    D. 15:2

49. What is the proper ratio of compressions to ventilations for two-rescuer adult CPR?

    A. 1:5

    B. 2:15

    C. 5:1

    D. 15:2

Chapter 7

Answers

1: **C.** The heart is a sensitive organ that is extremely dependent on oxygen. Arrhythmias develop quickly when the heart is deprived of oxygen. (ECTSI 5, p. 109)

2: **C.** Airway obstruction, respiratory arrest, and severe bleeding are all life-threatening emergencies that require immediate basic life support measures. (ECTSI 5, p. 110)

3: **B.** Like the heart, the brain is quite dependent on a continuous supply of oxygen. At normal body temperature, the brain is very likely to sustain permanent damage after as few as 6 minutes of being deprived of oxygen. (ECTSI 5, p. 111)

4: **B.** Ventricular fibrillation will not convert to a perfusing rhythm without defibrillation. However, the other conditions listed may respond to simple BLS intervention. (ECTSI 5, p. 159)

5: **A.** The appropriate course of action in this case is to roll the patient into a supine position keeping his head, neck, and back aligned, assess his ABCs, and begin basic life support if necessary. (ECTSI 5, p. 345)

6: **A.** Of the interventions listed, only the Heimlich maneuver is a BLS skill performed by EMTs. IV therapy, cardiac monitoring, and administration of medication are all ALS skills that require additional training outside the scope of practice of a basic EMT. (ECTSI 5, p. 122)

7: **D.** Living wills or advance directives are legal documents prepared in advance by the patient or the physician that provide directions regarding the patient's wishes concerning medical care. (ECTSI 5, p. 112)

8: **C.** When someone simply thinks that a living will exists, and there is no physical evidence of the document, the EMT is required to begin or continue treatment. In this situation, there are no legal grounds to stop resuscitation of the patient. (ECTSI 5, pp. 112–113)

9: **A.** The neighbor's opinion is just that, an opinion, and has no impact on this situation. Care is rendered under the concept of implied consent, that is, a life-threatening situation. You must assume that if the patient could, she would likely want care given and her life saved. (ECTSI 5, pp. 21–22)

Cardiopulmonary Resuscitation and Basic Life Support

10: **B.** The recovery position provides the patient with natural drainage of secretions, it does not block respiratory efforts, and it allows the EMT to monitor the patient carefully. (ECTSI 5, p. 113)

11: **D.** An unconscious adult loses the ability to protect the airway. The muscles of the throat and tongue relax and may fall back into the throat, causing airway obstruction. (ECTSI 5, p. 115)

12: **B.** The head-tilt maneuver is a simple technique that will very often open the airway. However, if the patient experienced traumatic injuries resulting in a possible cervical spine injury, this technique would be contraindicated. (ECTSI 5, p. 115)

13: **A.** A patient who is not breathing, but still has a pulse, needs only artificial ventilations to make sure the airway remains clear. If the patient has no pulse, CPR should be started. (ECTSI 5, p. 111)

14: **D.** Lividity, rigor mortis, and obvious putrefaction are all indications of certain death; therefore, CPR need not be started. A patient who has a head injury and is in cardiac arrest definitely needs CPR. (ECTSI 5, p. 112)

15: **B.** When you are alone with a patient who needs CPR, your first and most important action is to activate the EMS system to make sure that additional help is on the way. Without additional help, there is virtually no chance that the patient will survive. (ECTSI 5, p. 112)

16: **A.** Without physical evidence of a living will, it may as well not exist. CPR should be started immediately. If the living will turns up after resuscitation is in progress, medical control should be contacted and apprised of the situation. (ECTSI 5, p. 112)

17: **C.** CPR will not be effective if the patient is facedown, upright, or in a side-lying position. The patient should be supine and lying on a firm, flat surface. (ECTSI 5, p. 113)

18: **B.** The tongue relaxes and falls back into the airway when someone becomes unconscious. (ECTSI 5, p. 115)

19: **D.** Nasal flaring suggests respiratory distress, as the patient works and struggles to get more air. As such, it will not cause an airway obstruction. (ECTSI 5, p. 115)

20: **A.** Kneeling above the patient's head is the best position to perform the jaw-thrust maneuver without overexerting yourself or being uncomfortable. (ECTSI 5, p. 117)

Chapter 7

21: **B.** The patient must be deeply unconscious to tolerate the jaw-thrust maneuver. (ECTSI 5, p. 117)

22: **B.** Anoxia, or the absence of oxygen, is the end condition that produces biological death when a patient remains in respiratory arrest for more than 4 to 6 minutes. (ECTSI 5, p. 117)

23: **B.** Under normal circumstances, inspirations of less than 1 1/2 to 2 seconds would not be adequate for gas exchange to occur. (ECTSI 5, p. 117)

24: **A.** A rescuer breathing room air (21% oxygen) would use 5%, which would still leave a 16% oxygen in the exhaled air for the patient to breathe. (ECTSI 5, pp. 117–118)

25: **A.** Effective mouth-to-mask ventilation is characterized by the rise and fall of the patient's chest, feeling resistance of the lungs as they expand, and hearing and feeling air escape during exhalation. (ECTSI 5, p. 119)

26: **B.** A patient who has had a laryngectomy will have a stoma; therefore, mouth-to-stoma ventilations would be necessary. If any of the other techniques listed were used, the ventilations would enter the stomach with little or no air reaching the lungs. (ECTSI 5, p. 120)

27: **B.** During prolonged artificial ventilation, air will often move through the cardiac sphincter and enter the stomach, producing gastric distention. (ECTSI 5, p. 120)

28: **C.** Alveoli are air sacs in the lungs that receive the carbon dioxide that diffuses out of the blood. Therefore, alveoli are not likely to cause an airway obstruction. (ECTSI 5, p. 102)

29: **C.** When gastric distention occurs during artificial ventilation, the diaphragm is continually pushed upward, which reduces lung volume and makes regurgitation and possible aspiration more likely. (ECTSI 5, p. 120)

30: **A.** Sudden airway obstruction in adults often occurs during meals, and in many cases, alcohol is also a factor. (ECTSI 5, p. 121)

31: **B.** Grasping the throat is the universal sign of airway obstruction. With a complete obstruction, the patient cannot speak and obviously cannot exchange air, so the patient becomes cyanotic, not cold. (ECTSI 5, p. 121)

32: **C.** Currently, the two ways for an EMT-A to best manage airway obstruction in an adult is by providing abdominal thrusts to dislodge the foreign body, and then performing a finger sweep to remove the object. (ECTSI 5, p. 121)

Cardiopulmonary Resuscitation and Basic Life Support

33: **D.** With infants and children, a respiratory event typically precedes a cardiac event, because infants and children normally have no pathophysiologic reason for a major cardiac crisis. (ECTSI 5, p. 124)

34: **B.** The best way to open and maintain a child's airway is to use the chin-lift maneuver, making sure that neutral alignment of the cervical spine is maintained. (ECTSI 5, p. 125)

35: **B.** Ventilating a newborn infant once every 3 seconds or 20 times a minute is currently the recommended rate from the American Heart Association. (ECTSI 5, p. 126)

36: **D.** Pneumonia is not associated with upper airway obstruction, as it is a condition that affects the lung. (ECTSI 5, p. 470)

37: **D.** Ventricular fibrillation is the most common presenting rhythm for an adult in cardiac arrest, hence the importance of rapid defibrillation. (ECTSI 5, p. 144)

38: **B.** Ineffective cough, cyanosis signaling oxygen desaturation, and stridorous breathing are all serious signs of poor air exchange in a child. (ECTSI 5, p. 126)

39: **D.** Pulseless electrical activity (PEA) is a form of cardiac arrest in which the cardiac monitor shows adequate heart rate and rhythm, but there is no detectable pulse or blood pressure. (ECTSI 5, p. 144)

40: **D.** Placing your hand over the xiphoid process when performing chest compressions on an adult can result in laceration of abdominal organs, including the liver. Make sure you do not place your hands to the side of the sternum onto the ribs, as compressions in this area would likely result in fractured ribs. (ECTSI 5, p. 146)

41: **B.** Current thinking is that the ratio of compressions to contractions during adult CPR should be 1:1, or 50% compressions and 50% relaxations. This ratio is thought to provide the best potential for blood flow during CPR. (ECTSI 5, p. 146)

42: **A.** Check the pulse for 5 seconds after the first minute of CPR, and then every 5 minutes for as long as CPR continues. (ECTSI 5, p. 148)

43: **A.** "Perfect" CPR only produces 25% to 33% of the blood flow that the body produces normally. Therefore, extended periods without CPR (i.e., more than 5 seconds) can have serious adverse effects on the patient. (ECTSI 5, p. 151)

Chapter 7

44: **A.** Rapid defibrillation and IV access for cardiac medications are the structures built on the foundation of CPR. Without these additional therapies, the patient is not likely to survive. (ECTSI 5, pp. 144, 159–160)

45: **A.** The brachial pulse is the easiest to access and evaluate in infants. (ECTSI 5, p. 152)

46: **B.** Two finger compressions should be performed over the lower sternum on an infant in order to provide good blood flow and to reduce the likelihood of injury to any other structures. (ECTSI 5, p. 152)

47: **C.** Due to their naturally faster heart rate, the minimum compression rate for both infants and children is 100 compressions per minute. (ECTSI 5, p. 153)

48: **D.** The proper ratio of compressions to ventilations for one-rescuer adult CPR is 15:2. (ECTSI 5, p. 148)

49: **C.** The proper ratio of compressions to ventilations for two-rescuer adult CPR is 5:1. (ECTSI 5, p. 148)

Chapter 8

Airway Obstruction

Chapter Goals

The exercises in this chapter are designed to help the student to:

- identify commonly used devices for oxygen support.

- recognize signs and symptoms of airway obstruction.

- describe appropriate management of airway obstruction.

- identify suctioning devices and their appropriate use.

- recognize when supplemental oxygen is needed.

- describe the purpose of oropharyngeal and nasopharyngeal airways.

Chapter 8

Multiple-Choice Questions

Select the correct answer for each of the following questions. Each question has only *one* correct or best answer.

1. A patient's dentures should be left in during mouth-to-mouth resuscitation because the dentures may:

    A. be lost if they are removed.

    B. provide structure to the mouth.

    C. keep the patient from vomiting.

    D. control the ventilations enough to prevent distention.

2. When using an "S" tube, pocket mask, or other mouth-to-face breathing apparatus on an adult patient who is not breathing, you should provide:

    A. half-strength breaths.

    B. full-strength breaths.

    C. double-strength breaths.

    D. breaths four times the regular strength.

3. Oxygen can be dangerous because it:

    A. burns.

    B. explodes.

    C. supports combustion.

    D. may poison a patient if given too quickly.

4. What is the most common problem in using a bag-valve-mask device for administering supplemental oxygen?

    A. Overinflation of the lungs

    B. Failure to maintain the proper rate of ventilation

    C. Failure to make sure the bag fully inflates after each ventilation

    D. Failure to maintain an adequate seal around the nose and mouth

Airway Obstruction

5. Proper maintenance of oxygen cylinders includes:

   A. greasing the valves every month.

   B. storing the cylinder in a cool place.

   C. storing the cylinder on its side in a rack.

   D. ensuring a cylinder is completely empty before switching to a new one.

6. When ventilating a patient with a bag-valve-mask device, you should squeeze the bag until:

   A. it is empty.

   B. 100% oxygen is delivered.

   C. the patient's chest rises.

   D. the patient has spontaneous respirations.

7. After properly squeezing a bag-valve-mask device, you should:

   A. squeeze the bag again.

   B. allow the bag to reinflate.

   C. inflate the bag manually.

   D. remove the mask so the patient can exhale.

8. The curve of an oropharyngeal airway is first inserted upside down or sideways, and then inverted in order to:

   A. prevent the tongue from being pushed back.

   B. prevent the airway from damaging the teeth.

   C. allow the airway to conform to the tongue.

   D. allow the airway to conform to the shape of the mouth.

Chapter 8

9. Of the following, which device will deliver the highest concentration of oxygen?

   A. Venturi mask

   B. Nasal cannula

   C. Simple face mask

   D. Nonrebreathing face mask with a reservoir bag

10. The first step in giving supplemental oxygen with a demand valve resuscitator is to:

    A. seal the mask to the patient's face.

    B. place the patient in the coma position.

    C. elevate the head of the stretcher.

    D. make sure an oropharyngeal airway has been inserted.

11. A patient begins to gag and retch during insertion of an oropharyngeal airway. You should immediately:

    A. remove the airway and be ready for the patient to vomit.

    B. remove the airway and insert a shorter one.

    C. pull it out slightly, as it was inserted too deeply.

    D. pull it out and reinsert it, as it was not inserted correctly.

12. You are providing ventilation with a bag-valve-mask device. To enrich the oxygen supply, attach the oxygen tubing to the mask, and then adjust the flow rate to:

    A. 4 L/min.

    B. 6 L/min.

    C. 8 L/min.

    D. the highest flow rate possible.

Airway Obstruction

13. After inflating the reservoir bag of a face mask, the oxygen flow rate should be:

    A. set and maintained at 2 to 4 L/min.

    B. set and maintained at 6 to 8 L/min.

    C. adjusted so the reservoir is fully inflated.

    D. adjusted so the reservoir neither completely collapses nor is fully inflated.

14. A patient who appears to have a locked mandible is not breathing. The most appropriate way to ventilate this patient is with the:

    A. "S" tube.

    B. chest pressure method.

    C. mouth-to-nose technique.

    D. back pressure-arm lift method.

15. A patient in respiratory arrest should not be suctioned any longer than:

    A. 2 seconds.

    B. 5 seconds.

    C. 10 seconds.

    D. 15 seconds.

16. Which of the following statements about opening the airway of a small child is true?

    A. A child's neck is less flexible than an adult's neck.

    B. A child's head should be tilted back as far as possible.

    C. A child's airway is likely to collapse if the head is tilted back too far.

    D. A child's tongue is more likely to obstruct the airway than an adult's tongue.

Chapter 8

17. You and your partner arrive at the scene of an automobile accident in which an unconscious man is found in a sitting position in the driver's seat. He does not appear to be breathing. While you can reach the patient, he cannot be removed from the car right away. The first step in caring for this patient should be to:

    A. attempt extrication with a pry bar and then move the patient so you can begin assessing his ABCs.

    B. begin ventilation with a mechanical pressure-cycled resuscitator as your partner begins extrication.

    C. perform a thorough examination, since he cannot be moved until a full assessment has been made.

    D. support the patient in an upright position, perform the chin-lift maneuver with the face supported and looking forward, and begin ventilation as your partner begins extrication.

18. Excessive volume in infant ventilation may cause:

    A. collapse of the trachea.

    B. rupture of the diaphragm.

    C. injury to the lungs.

    D. hemothorax.

19. The most common causes of airway obstruction in unconscious patients are fluids in the airway and:

    A. pieces of food.

    B. debris from injury.

    C. false teeth or bridgework.

    D. the tongue falling back into the throat.

Airway Obstruction

20. An unconscious woman who sounds like she is snoring as she breathes most likely has:

    A. a spasm of the larynx.

    B. a spasm of the bronchi.

    C. a partial airway obstruction.

    D. foreign matter in the lungs.

21. You are resuscitating a patient with a bag-valve-mask device. The patient's chest does not rise when the bag is squeezed. You should:

    A. squeeze the bag harder.

    B. squeeze the bag easier.

    C. change the mask on the device.

    D. make a tighter seal with the device.

22. The best way to determine whether a child needs supplemental oxygen is to assess the child's:

    A. respirations.

    B. blood pressure.

    C. pupillary reaction.

    D. level of comfort with and without supplemental oxygen.

23. An unconscious patient with a complete airway obstruction should be:

    A. placed in a coma position.

    B. given a series of abdominal thrusts.

    C. given supplemental oxygen immediately.

    D. intubated with an oropharyngeal airway.

Chapter 8

24. A simple face mask that delivers 8 to 12 liters of oxygen per minute provides approximately how much oxygen?

    A. 15% to 20%

    B. 35% to 60%

    C. 75% to 90%

    D. 100%

25. A patient in cardiac arrest should be given supplemental oxygen at:

    A. 50%.

    B. 75%.

    C. 80%.

    D. 100%.

26. The proper length of an oropharyngeal airway can be estimated as the distance between the:

    A. nose and chin.

    B. chin and earlobe.

    C. corner of the eye and chin.

    D. corner of the mouth and earlobe.

27. Extreme caution should be used when inserting a nasopharyngeal airway into a patient with severe head or facial trauma, because the airway may:

    A. cause vomiting.

    B. penetrate the cranium.

    C. injure the hard palate.

    D. cause additional soft tissue damage.

Airway Obstruction

28. What is the principal difference between a D cylinder and an M cylinder?

    A. The D cylinder contains more oxygen.

    B. The D cylinder has a threaded gas outlet.

    C. The M cylinder serves as the main supply on ambulances.

    D. The M cylinder has a valve that accepts a yoke-type pressure-reducing gauge.

29. Humidification of supplemental oxygen is important because the extremely dry oxygen that leaves the cylinder will:

    A. dry the patient's mucous membranes.

    B. damage the flowmeter at high flow rates.

    C. be too oxygen rich and could poison the patient.

    D. evaporate as soon as it comes in contact with the atmosphere.

30. To deliver oxygen at 100%, you would most likely select which of the following devices?

    A. Nasal cannula

    B. Simple face mask

    C. Venturi mask

    D. Bag-valve-mask device with a reservoir bag

Chapter 8

Answers

1: **B.** Dentures should be left in during mouth-to-mouth resuscitation in order to provide structure to the mouth. (ECTSI 5, p. 116)

2: **B.** Regardless of the device used, you should supply full-strength breaths while ventilating a patient. (ECTSI 5, pp. 168–169)

3: **C.** While oxygen itself does not burn or explode, it does support combustion. (ECTSI 5, p. 177)

4: **D.** The most common problem when using a bag-valve-mask device is that the operator does not obtain an adequate seal. (ECTSI 5, p. 174)

5: **B.** Proper maintenance of oxygen cylinders includes storing the cylinder in a cool place. Never apply grease or any lubricant to the valves of the cylinder. (ECTSI 5, p. 179)

6: **C.** In ventilating a patient with a bag-valve-mask device, you should squeeze the bag until the patient's chest rises. (ECTSI 5, p. 174)

7: **B.** After squeezing the bag of a bag-valve-mask device, you should release the bag and allow it to reinflate. (ECTSI 5, p. 174)

8: **A.** An oropharyngeal airway is inserted upside down or sideways, then inverted in order to prevent the tongue from being pushed back. (ECTSI 5, p. 170)

9: **D.** A nonrebreathing face mask with a reservoir bag will deliver up to 95% oxygen. (ECTSI 5, p. 183)

10: **D.** Before giving supplemental oxygen with a demand valve resuscitator, you should ensure that an oropharyngeal airway is inserted to prevent the tongue from blocking the airway. (ECTSI 5, pp. 184–185, 807)

11: **A.** You should immediately remove an oropharyngeal airway if the patient begins to gag or makes any effort to fight insertion of the airway. This will reduce the possibility that the patient will vomit and possibly aspirate the vomitus. (ECTSI 5, pp. 170, 807)

12: **D.** To enrich the oxygen supply, use the highest flow rate possible. (ECTSI 5, p. 174)

13: **D.** When using a face mask with a reservoir bag, the flow rate should be adjusted so that the bag neither fully inflates nor collapses as the patient breathes. (ECTSI 5, p. 183)

Airway Obstruction

14: **C.** If a patient who has a locked mandible is not breathing, you should attempt to ventilate using the mouth-to-nose method. (ECTSI 5, p. 119)

15: **B.** Since ventilation must be interrupted, suctioning should not be used for more than 5 seconds. (ECTSI 5, p. 151)

16: **C.** Because the cartilage that supports the trachea is not fully developed in an infant or small child, hyperextending the neck may cause the airway to collapse. (ECTSI 5, p. 125)

17: **D.** The first step in caring for this patient is to address ventilation. Therefore, you should support the patient in an upright position, perform the chin-lift maneuver with the face supported and looking forward, and begin ventilation. Your partner can then concentrate on extrication. (ECTSI 5, pp. 706–709)

18: **C.** Excessive volume during artificial ventilation of an infant can result in injury to the lungs. (ECTSI 5, pp. 125–126)

19: **D.** The most common causes of airway obstruction in unconscious patients are fluids in the airway and the tongue falling back into the throat. (ECTSI 5, p. 115)

20: **C.** Snoring sounds during breathing indicate a partial obstruction of the airway. (ECTSI 5, p. 124)

21: **D.** The most common failure when attempting to ventilate a patient with a bag-valve-mask device is failing to maintain a tight seal around the patient's nose and mouth. Therefore, you should attempt to make a tighter seal with the device. (ECTSI 5, p. 174)

22: **D.** If you are unsure about whether to give a child supplemental oxygen, you should give the oxygen and then judge the patient's reaction. (ECTSI 5, pp. 177–178)

23: **B.** An unconscious patient with a complete airway obstruction should be given a series of abdominal thrusts. (ECTSI 5, p. 121)

24: **B.** A simple face mask with a flow rate of 8 to 12 L/min delivers approximately 35% to 60% oxygen. (ECTSI 5, p. 182)

25: **D.** Any patient in cardiac arrest should be given supplemental oxygen at 100%. (ECTSI 5, p. 168)

Chapter 8

26: **D.** The proper length of an oropharyngeal airway can be estimated as the distance between the corner of the mouth and the earlobe. (ECTSI 5, p. 171)

27: **B.** Use extreme care when inserting a nasopharyngeal airway into a patient with severe head or facial trauma to avoid penetrating the cranium. (ECTSI 5, p. 173)

28: **C.** The M cylinder is used as the main oxygen supply tank on ambulances and can hold 3,000 liters of oxygen. (ECTSI 5, p. 178)

29: **A.** Humidification of oxygen is an important consideration in administering supplemental oxygen, as the extremely dry oxygen leaving the cylinder can dry the patient's mucous membranes and interfere with respiration. (ECTSI 5, p. 180)

30: **D.** Of the choices listed, the bag-valve-mask device with a reservoir bag delivers oxygen at concentrations approaching 100%. (ECTSI 5, p. 184)

Chapter 9

Control of Bleeding and Shock

Chapter Goals

The exercises in this chapter are designed to help the student to:

- recognize the significance of bleeding.

- explain how to control bleeding using direct pressure.

- identify other methods for controlling bleeding.

- describe how to manage epistaxis.

- recognize the signs and symptoms of shock.

- describe basic measures for treatment of shock.

Chapter 9

Multiple-Choice Questions

Select the correct answer for each of the following questions. Each question has only *one* correct or best answer.

1. Of the following, which is the most serious complication of internal bleeding?

    A. Myocardial infarction

    B. Hypovolemic shock

    C. Cardiogenic shock

    D. Collapse of the lungs

2. A conscious person in shock should be given:

    A. clear liquids.

    B. coffee or tea.

    C. fluids with special electrolytes.

    D. nothing by mouth.

3. Arterial bleeding is characterized by:

    A. bright red blood flowing steadily from the wound.

    B. bright red blood spurting from the wound.

    C. dark maroon blood flowing steadily from the wound.

    D. dark maroon blood spurting from the wound.

4. The best way to control bleeding from an extremity is with:

    A. a tourniquet and elevation.

    B. direct pressure and elevation.

    C. pressure on arterial pulse points.

    D. bandaging.

Control of Bleeding and Shock

5. Treatment of a nosebleed should include:

    A. placing the patient in a side-lying position.

    B. applying pressure by squeezing the nostrils.

    C. applying pressure on the carotid arteries.

    D. giving the patient aspirin for clotting purposes.

6. Signs of internal bleeding include:

    A. increased pulse rate and warm skin.

    B. increased pulse rate and clammy skin.

    C. reduced pulse rate and dilated pupils.

    D. reduced pulse rate and a soft abdomen.

7. To appropriately record the time a tourniquet is applied, you must:

    A. call medical control immediately after application.

    B. write "applied at" and the time on the tourniquet once it has been applied.

    C. write the time of application in the patient's medical record at the hospital.

    D. mark TK and the time of application on tape and place it on the patient's forehead.

8. Which of the following signs and symptoms suggest possible hypovolemic shock?

    A. Slow, strong pulse, dizziness, cold perspiration, nausea

    B. Weak, rapid pulse, cold, clammy skin, pallor, shallow breathing

    C. Blank expression, cold extremities, regular breathing

    D. Blank expression, chills, unconsciousness, dry skin

9. The first step in caring for a patient in shock is to:

    A. give the patient water to drink.

    B. help the patient to lie down and elevate the legs.

    C. place blankets under and over the patient.

    D. check for an open airway and then administer oxygen.

Chapter 9

10. A man has an open, bleeding gash on his forehead after an automobile accident. To control the bleeding, you should apply:

    A. pressure to the carotid artery.

    B. pressure to the subclavian artery.

    C. a sterile dressing with a loose bandage.

    D. a sterile dressing with a snug bandage.

11. A man is cut above the ankle by a lawn mower blade. If the bleeding cannot be controlled with direct pressure, you should apply pressure on which of the following arteries?

    A. Dorsalis pedis

    B. Subclavian

    C. Temporal

    D. Femoral

12. You cannot control bleeding with direct or arterial pressure in a patient who has an amputated leg. You should next:

    A. irrigate the stump with sterile water.

    B. prepare to transport the patient immediately.

    C. apply a tourniquet about 2 inches above the stump.

    D. apply warm compresses and a loose dressing over the stump.

13. A patient who has lost a massive amount of blood should be given oxygen at:

    A. 25%.

    B. 50%.

    C. 80%.

    D. 100%.

Control of Bleeding and Shock

14. A patient who has severe traumatic injuries should be treated for shock:

    A. after all other problems are treated.

    B. only when all signs and symptoms of shock appear.

    C. only when a pattern of signs and symptoms develops.

    D. routinely without waiting for signs or symptoms to develop.

15. Which of the following deteriorates the fastest without constant perfusion?

    A. Lungs

    B. Liver

    C. Kidneys

    D. Skeletal muscle

16. Psychogenic shock or fainting occurs because the blood supply to the brain is:

    A. under too much pressure.

    B. deoxygenated.

    C. oxygen saturated.

    D. suddenly and sharply reduced.

17. Which of the following is a sign of anaphylactic shock?

    A. Constricted pupils

    B. Cool, moist skin

    C. Difficulty breathing

    D. Epistaxis

18. Of the following, the only really effective treatment the EMT can provide to a patient in anaphylactic shock is:

    A. immersion in an ice bath.

    B. administration of 100% oxygen.

    C. vigorous massage of the extremities.

    D. an intracardiac injection of epinephrine.

Chapter 9

19. A conscious patient in cardiogenic shock should be transported in what position?

    A. Coma

    B. Prone

    C. Semisitting

    D. Trendelenburg's

20. Which of the following devices may be used as a tourniquet?

    A. Belt

    B. Rope

    C. Blood pressure cuff

    D. Narrow strip of bandage

21. Use of a tourniquet to stop bleeding from an extremity should be considered a measure of last resort because a tourniquet:

    A. is painful.

    B. does not always work.

    C. may cause loss of the limb.

    D. may become loose after an extended period.

22. Although any place where a blood vessel can be pressed against a bony surface is considered a pressure point, the two most commonly used are located at the:

    A. neck and the groin.

    B. medial upper arm and the groin.

    C. medial upper arm and the medial thigh.

    D. posterior upper arm and the medial thigh.

Control of Bleeding and Shock

23. Venous bleeding is characterized by:

    A. bright red blood flowing steadily from the wound.

    B. bright red blood spurting from the wound.

    C. dark maroon blood flowing steadily from the wound.

    D. dark maroon blood spurting from the wound.

24. What type of shock is most likely to cause swelling of the face, tongue, and respiratory tract?

    A. Septic

    B. Metabolic

    C. Anaphylactic

    D. Hypovolemic

25. Which of the following arteries is the **LEAST** dependable for taking a pulse in a patient who appears to be in shock?

    A. Carotid

    B. Radial

    C. Femoral

    D. Brachial

26. Which of the following arteries is the most dependable for taking a pulse?

    A. Radial

    B. Carotid

    C. Brachial

    D. Dorsalis pedis

Chapter 9

27. A patient has severe bleeding from a chest wound, and no dressing or bandage is available. The most appropriate action in this case would be to:

    A. use a pressure point.

    B. use your gloved hand to apply direct pressure.

    C. quickly try to find a bandage, clean cloth, or sanitary napkin.

    D. wash your bare hand with soap and then apply direct pressure.

28. Control of severe hemorrhage should be:

    A. considered a high priority of treatment.

    B. considered critical only if the patient has a weak pulse and low blood pressure.

    C. attempted only after a full survey of the patient.

    D. attempted only if you have access to gloves and some form of dressing.

29. What type of shock results from an injury to or a failure of the nervous system?

    A. Hemorrhagic

    B. Neurogenic

    C. Psychogenic

    D. Anaphylactic

30. Once a tourniquet has been applied, it must be:

    A. removed after 1 hour.

    B. tightened and left on until removed by a physician.

    C. tightened for 20 minutes and released for 10 minutes.

    D. tightened for 10 minutes and released for 10 minutes.

31. What type of shock results from an inadequate oxygen supply?

    A. Hemorrhagic

    B. Respiratory

    C. Metabolic

    D. Neurogenic

Control of Bleeding and Shock

32. To help a patient in shock maintain adequate blood flow and oxygen supply to the brain, you should:

    A. tilt the entire body up at the head.

    B. slightly elevate the upper part of the body.

    C. elevate the lower extremities.

    D. elevate the lower extremities and trunk of the body.

33. What type of shock can result from the loss of 2 pints of blood in a 30-year-old man of average weight and height?

    A. Septic

    B. Metabolic

    C. Cardiogenic

    D. Hypovolemic

34. The use of oxygen in treatment of shock is considered to be:

    A. a routine part of treatment.

    B. of no particular benefit to the patient.

    C. useful only if the patient has difficulty breathing.

    D. a last resort measure if all other treatment fails.

35. In emergency medicine, the term *shock* is defined as:

    A. sudden hemorrhage.

    B. a cardiovascular accident.

    C. emptying of the blood vessels.

    D. collapse of the cardiovascular system.

36. Neurogenic shock is often a result of damage to the:

    A. lungs.

    B. heart.

    C. spinal cord.

    D. immune system.

Chapter 9

Answers

1: **B.** The most serious complication of internal bleeding is hypovolemic shock. (ECTSI 5, p. 292)

2: **D.** A conscious patient in shock should be given nothing by mouth. (ECTSI 5, p. 213)

3: **B.** Arterial bleeding is characterized by bright red blood that spurts with each contraction of the heart. (ECTSI 5, pp. 189–190)

4: **B.** The best way to control bleeding from an extremity, and the least damaging, is to use direct pressure and elevation. (ECTSI 5, p. 191)

5: **B.** You should squeeze the nostrils of a patient with a nosebleed. (ECTSI 5, p. 199)

6: **B.** An increased pulse rate and clammy skin suggest possible internal bleeding. (ECTSI 5, p. 200)

7: **D.** After you apply a tourniquet, you must fasten a piece of tape to the patient's forehead and mark TK and the time of application. (ECTSI 5, p. 198)

8: **B.** Hypovolemic shock is characterized by a weak, rapid pulse; cold, clammy skin; pallor; and shallow, often irregular respirations. (ECTSI 5, p. 212)

9: **D.** The first step in caring for a patient in shock is to check for an open airway and then administer oxygen. (ECTSI 5, p. 212)

10: **D.** Bleeding from a head wound should be treated with a sterile dressing bandage applied snug enough to control the bleeding. (ECTSI 5, p. 330)

11: **D.** Since the bleeding is above the ankle, you should use the femoral pressure point, which is proximal to the wound. (ECTSI 5, p. 193)

12: **C.** In this situation, a tourniquet should be applied about 2 inches above the stump. (ECTSI 5, p. 196)

13: **D.** You should administer oxygen at 100% to compensate for the loss of oxygen-carrying red blood cells. (ECTSI 5, pp. 177, 202, 216)

14: **D.** Patients with severe traumatic injuries should be treated for shock routinely to prevent the onset of shock. (ECTSI 5, p. 228)

Control of Bleeding and Shock

15: **A.** The lungs need constant perfusion in order to function properly, and will deteriorate much quicker than the other structures listed. (ECTSI 5, pp. 134–135)

16: **D.** Psychogenic shock or fainting usually occurs because the blood supply to the brain is suddenly and sharply reduced. (ECTSI 5, p. 209)

17: **C.** Difficulty breathing or dyspnea is a common sign of anaphylactic shock. (ECTSI 5, p. 211)

18: **B.** Since anaphylaxis can only be effectively treated by drug therapy, you can provide only supportive treatment with 100% oxygen. (ECTSI 5, p. 216)

19: **C.** A conscious patient in cardiogenic shock should be transported in a semisitting position and given oxygen. (ECTSI 5, pp. 214–215)

20: **C.** Of the items listed, only the blood pressure cuff is appropriate for use as a tourniquet. (ECTSI 5, pp. 196–197)

21: **C.** A tourniquet, if left on for an extended period, can cause the loss of the portion of the limb distal to it. (ECTSI 5, p. 196)

22: **B.** The two most effective pressure points are located at the brachial and femoral arteries, located inside the upper arm and at the groin. (ECTSI 5, p. 63)

23: **C.** Venous bleeding is characteristically dark red and flows steadily from a wound. (ECTSI 5, p. 190)

24: **C.** Swelling of the face, tongue, and respiratory tract are all signs of anaphylactic shock. (ECTSI 5, p. 211)

25: **B.** The radial artery, while most commonly used, is the least reliable since it is most distal from the heart and is small in diameter. (ECTSI 5, p. 67)

26: **B.** The carotid artery is the most reliable for taking a pulse. (ECTSI 5, p. 67)

27: **B.** Use your gloved hand to apply direct pressure. Do not waste valuable time washing or looking for a dressing of any kind. (ECTSI 5, p. 375)

28: **A.** Control of hemorrhage is always given one of the highest priorities of treatment. (ECTSI 5, p. 189)

Chapter 9

29: **B.** Neurogenic shock is caused by an injury to or a failure of the nervous system. (ECTSI 5, p. 209)

30: **B.** If a tourniquet must be used, it must be put on tightly, left on, and be removed only by a physician. (ECTSI 5, pp. 196–198)

31: **B.** Respiratory shock is caused by an inadequate oxygen supply. (ECTSI 5, p. 211)

32: **C.** Elevation of the lower extremities increases the amount of blood available to the chest and head. (ECTSI 5, p. 213)

33: **D.** Hypovolemic shock results from excessive blood loss. (ECTSI 5, p. 210)

34: **A.** Oxygen should be given to all patients in shock. (ECTSI 5, p. 213)

35: **D.** Shock is defined as a collapse of the cardiovascular system resulting in inadequate tissue perfusion. (ECTSI 5, p. 206)

36: **C.** Neurogenic shock is often a result of damage to the spinal cord. (ECTSI 5, p. 209)

Chapter 10
Wounds and Bandaging

Chapter Goals

The exercises in this chapter are designed to help the student to:

- identify the characteristics of closed and open wounds.

- describe the purposes of dressing and bandaging wounds.

- identify appropriate materials for dressing and bandaging wounds.

- describe appropriate methods for dressing and bandaging wounds.

Chapter 10

Multiple-Choice Questions

Select the correct answer for each of the following questions. Each question has only *one* correct or best answer.

1. A bandage should be applied so that it:

    A. just covers the dressing.

    B. is loose enough to allow air to enter.

    C. extends 8 to 12 inches beyond the dressing on each side.

    D. extends enough beyond the dressing to prevent dirt from reaching the wound or dressing.

2. A pressure bandage is applied to a patient's leg, but the bleeding has not stopped. Your next step would be to:

    A. apply pressure on the proper pressure point.

    B. apply pressure to the bandage with your gloved hand or tighten it, taking care so that it will not turn into a tourniquet.

    C. tighten the bandage so it becomes a tourniquet.

    D. place another bandage 6 inches above the wound.

3. Possible contamination of an open wound can be avoided if you make sure that:

    A. dressings are stacked to control bleeding, not removed and replaced.

    B. constant pressure is placed on the wound.

    C. all dirt, grass, and debris is removed from the wound.

    D. the wound is thoroughly cleansed before the dressing is applied.

4. When bandaging an extremity, you should ensure that the bandage is applied:

    A. tightly over the fingers or toes.

    B. loosely over the fingers or toes.

    C. so the fingers or toes are exposed.

    D. so the fingers or toes are exposed, but completely immobilized.

Wounds and Bandaging

5. What is the proper sequence for treating an open wound of an extremity?

    A. Elevate the extremity, and then apply a sterile dressing and bandage.

    B. Apply a sterile compression dressing, immobilize the extremity, then elevate the extremity.

    C. Wash the wound, apply a sterile dressing and bandage, then elevate the extremity.

    D. Wash the wound, apply a sterile dressing and bandage, then immobilize the extremity.

6. Of the following, which would be most appropriate for stabilizing an impaled object?

    A. Elastic bandage

    B. Roller bandage

    C. Occlusive dressing

    D. Absorbent cotton

7. Which of the following statements about dressings and bandages is **FALSE**?

    A. Bandages need not be sterile.

    B. Bandages are used to hold dressings in place.

    C. Dressings are used to hold bandages in place.

    D. Dressings are used to prevent contamination.

8. After applying both a dressing and a bandage to a laceration below the elbow, you should check for changes in sensation in the patient's:

    A. fingers.

    B. shoulder.

    C. elbow.

    D. neck.

Chapter 10

9. If blood soaks through a dressing, you should:

    A. replace it with a new one.

    B. apply pressure with your bare hand.

    C. remove the dressing and compress a pressure point.

    D. place another dressing on top of the first one.

10. A bandage may be applied in generally the same way to both the elbow and the:

    A. hand.

    B. knee.

    C. foot.

    D. shoulder.

11. A small laceration can be covered properly with:

    A. an occlusive dressing.

    B. a self-adhering dressing.

    C. a universal dressing.

    D. an elastic bandage.

12. An occlusive dressing is most commonly used on a:

    A. laceration.

    B. puncture wound

    C. sucking chest wound.

    D. closed comminuted fracture.

13. After wetting a dressing with sterile saline solution, the "wound field" is considered:

    A. aseptic.

    B. sterile.

    C. antimicrobial.

    D. open to contamination.

Wounds and Bandaging

14. The use of cotton as a dressing is not recommended because:

    A. its fibers can become stuck to the wound.

    B. its absorbency varies depending on the type of injury.

    C. it is too expensive to keep well stocked.

    D. it is impossible to keep sterile.

15. What is the proper sequence for treating a swollen closed soft tissue injury to the leg?

    A. Cold, compression, elevation, and then splinting

    B. Compression, elevation, cold, and then splinting

    C. Elevation, cold, compression, and then splinting

    D. Elevation, compression, cold, and then splinting

16. An avulsion is an injury in which:

    A. there is snagging and tearing of tissue.

    B. a flap of skin and tissue is hanging or torn loose.

    C. a sharp, pointed object has disrupted the skin and underlying tissue.

    D. the skin surface is abraded with penetration of all layers of the skin.

17. Which of the following is considered a closed injury?

    A. Avulsion

    B. Puncture

    C. Laceration

    D. Contusion

Chapter 10

18. Appropriate care of an amputated part should include:

    A. carefully replacing the part at its original site, applying a dressing, and then bandaging firmly.

    B. carefully replacing the part at its original site, and then securing it with moist dressings and bandages.

    C. placing the part in a cold, sterile saline solution, and then transporting it with the patient.

    D. wrapping the part in sterile gauze, placing it in a plastic bag in a cool container, and then transporting it with the patient.

19. A patient has a knife protruding from an abdominal wound. The appropriate course of action is to:

    A. remove it, to prevent infection.

    B. remove it, to prevent it from going deeper.

    C. remove it, to apply a pressure dressing.

    D. leave it, because removal may cause serious bleeding.

20. An open wound characterized by capillary bleeding is called:

    A. an abrasion.

    B. an avulsion.

    C. a contusion.

    D. a laceration.

21. A collection of blood in the tissues resulting from injury or a broken blood vessel is called:

    A. an incision.

    B. an abrasion.

    C. an avulsion.

    D. a hematoma.

Wounds and Bandaging

22. Swelling and bleeding in a severe closed soft tissue injury can be controlled by applying:

    A. direct pressure and then elevating.

    B. cold and transporting immediately.

    C. cold and a snug bandage for mild pressure.

    D. warmth and a snug bandage for mild pressure.

23. Which of the following injuries is most susceptible to tetanus?

    A. Laceration

    B. Amputation

    C. Incision

    D. Puncture

24. Formation of an air embolism in the brain may result from a:

    A. laceration of the femoral artery.

    B. laceration of the jugular vein.

    C. soft tissue injury.

    D. femoral fracture.

25. Which of the following is considered an open wound?

    A. Contusion

    B. Hematoma

    C. Laceration

    D. Ecchymosis

26. Which of the following wounds is characterized by jagged skin edges and penetration to underlying muscles?

    A. Laceration

    B. Abrasion

    C. Incision

    D. Puncture

Chapter 10

27. What type of soft tissue injury is caused by the impact of a blunt object?

   A. Contusion

   B. Concussion

   C. Comminuted

   D. Avulsion

Answers

1: **D.** A bandage should extend enough beyond the dressing to prevent dirt from reaching the wound or dressing. (ECTSI 5, p. 191)

2: **B.** If bleeding does not stop after a pressure bandage has been applied, apply pressure on the bandage with your gloved hand or tighten it, ensuring that it does not impair circulation. (ECTSI 5, p. 191)

3: **A.** You can avoid possible contamination of an open wound if dressings are stacked, not removed and replaced, in the attempt to control bleeding. (ECTSI 5, p. 217)

4: **C.** You should leave the patient's fingers and toes exposed to continually monitor circulation. (ECTSI 5, p. 242)

5: **B.** The proper sequence for treating an open wound of an extremity is as follows: apply a sterile compression dressing; immobilize the extremity; then elevate the extremity. (ECTSI 5, p. 237)

6: **B.** Of the choices given, a roller bandage is best for stabilizing an impaled object. (ECTSI 5, pp. 239–240)

7: **C.** The statement, "Dressings are used to hold bandages in place," is incorrect. (ECTSI 5, p. 242)

8: **A.** Once the dressing and bandage are applied, check for changes in sensation in the patient's fingers to ensure circulation is not impaired. (ECTSI 5, p. 242)

9: **D.** If a dressing becomes soaked with blood, place another on top of it without removing the original dressing. (ECTSI 5, p. 237)

10: **B.** An elbow and a knee are bandaged generally the same way. (ECTSI 5, pp. 293, 307)

Wounds and Bandaging

11: **B.** A small laceration can be covered properly with a self-adhering dressing. (ECTSI 5, p. 241)

12: **C.** An occlusive dressing is most commonly used to seal a sucking chest wound. (ECTSI 5, p. 242)

13: **D.** The "wound field" is open to contamination once it has been moistened with saline solution. (ECTSI 5, p. 237)

14: **A.** Cotton is not recommended for use as a dressing because its fibers can become stuck to the wound. (ECTSI 5, p. 406)

15: **A.** The proper sequence for treating a closed soft tissue wound to the leg is as follows: apply cold, compression, elevation, and then splint. (ECTSI 5, p. 234)

16: **B.** An avulsion injury is characterized by a flap of skin or tissue torn off or left hanging. (ECTSI 5, p. 235)

17: **D.** A contusion is a closed soft tissue injury, while avulsions, punctures, and lacerations are all open wounds. (ECTSI 5, p. 234)

18: **D.** An amputated part should be wrapped in sterile gauze, placed in a plastic bag inside a cool container, and then transported with the patient. (ECTSI 5, p. 238)

19: **D.** In this case, the impaled object should not be removed. Removal could cause further tissue damage and increased bleeding. (ECTSI 5, p. 239)

20: **A.** An abrasion or "scrape" usually covers a larger area than other kinds of wounds and is characterized by capillary bleeding. (ECTSI 5, p. 235)

21: **D.** A hematoma is pooling of blood under the skin caused when vessels are disrupted without the skin being broken or punctured. (ECTSI 5, p. 234)

22: **C.** Cold should be applied to reduce swelling and a snug bandage applied. If the injury is to an extremity, it should also be immobilized. (ECTSI 5, p. 234)

23: **D.** Puncture wounds are most susceptible to tetanus due to their depth and usual lack of bleeding. (ECTSI 5, p. 236)

24: **B.** An air embolism in the brain can result from a laceration of the jugular vein. (ECTSI 5, p. 640)

25: **C.** A laceration is considered an open wound. (ECTSI 5, p. 235)

Chapter 10

26: **A.** A laceration has jagged edges while an incision has straight, clean edges. Both can bleed freely. (ECTSI 5, p. 235)

27: **A.** A contusion is a soft tissue injury caused by the force of a blunt object. (ECTSI 5, p. 234)

Chapter 11

The Musculoskeletal System

Chapter Goals

The exercises in this chapter are designed to help the student to:

- describe the differences between voluntary and involuntary muscles.

- explain how muscle is attached to bone and how this provides for body movement.

- describe the functions of the skeletal system.

- describe the various types of bone joints.

- explain the differences between fractures, sprains, strains, and dislocations.

Chapter 11

Multiple-Choice Questions

Select the correct answer for each of the following questions. Each question has only *one* correct or best answer.

1. Bones are able to move because they are attached to:

    A. tubular muscles.

    B. smooth muscles.

    C. voluntary muscles.

    D. involuntary muscles.

2. The distal point at which skeletal muscle attaches to the bone is called its:

    A. origin.

    B. insertion.

    C. opposition.

    D. articulation.

3. The bone that connects with the femur at the knee is called the:

    A. tibia.

    B. fibula.

    C. radius.

    D. humerus.

4. The most commonly fractured ribs are the:

    A. first through fifth.

    B. second through fourth.

    C. fifth through tenth.

    D. eleventh and twelfth.

The Musculoskeletal System

5. Which of the following bones connects to the humerus?

   A. Tibia

   B. Radius

   C. Fibula

   D. Clavicle

6. The flat, bony structure that joins the ribs at the front of the chest is called the:

   A. scapula.

   B. clavicle.

   C. sternum.

   D. xiphoid process.

7. The jaw is made up of what two bones?

   A. Clavicle and zygoma

   B. Maxilla and clavicle

   C. Maxilla and mandible

   D. Zygoma and temporal

8. A dislocation is an injury to:

   A. a joint.

   B. a bone.

   C. tendons.

   D. a muscle.

9. The function of synovial fluid is to:

   A. produce red blood cells.

   B. lubricate the bones at a joint.

   C. protect the brain and spinal cord.

   D. ensure that breathing is automatic.

Chapter 11

10. The function of involuntary muscle is to:

    A. help prevent muscle cramps.

    B. allow for movement at a joint.

    C. respond to commands from the brain.

    D. carry out the automatic work of the body.

11. When skeletal muscle is stimulated by nerves, it will:

    A. extend.

    B. expand.

    C. contract.

    D. revolve.

12. The biceps is composed of what type of muscle tissue?

    A. Cardiac

    B. Smooth

    C. Voluntary

    D. Involuntary

13. The diaphragm is unique in that it is both a:

    A. smooth and striated muscle.

    B. cardiac and voluntary muscle.

    C. smooth and voluntary muscle.

    D. voluntary and involuntary muscle.

14. The muscles of the blood vessel walls are considered to be:

    A. striated.

    B. voluntary.

    C. peripheral.

    D. involuntary.

The Musculoskeletal System

15. The knee joint is considered to be what type of joint?

    A. Hinge

    B. Rotating

    C. Revolving

    D. Ball-and-socket

16. Which of the following structures heals itself by forming more of itself?

    A. Skeletal muscle

    B. Smooth muscle

    C. Bone

    D. Cardiac muscle

17. Of the following, in which area is a dislocation most likely to occur?

    A. Patella

    B. Sacroiliac

    C. Trochanter

    D. Sternoclavicular joint

18. Which of the following is an example of involuntary muscle?

    A. Triceps

    B. Deltoid

    C. Intestine wall

    D. Xiphoid process

19. Ball-and-socket joints allow motion:

    A. from front to back.

    B. from side to side.

    C. in all directions.

    D. in one direction.

Chapter 11

20. What material covers the ends of bones in joints where motion occurs?

    A. Periosteum

    B. Compact bone

    C. Cancellous bone

    D. Articular cartilage

21. Patients with injuries to bones and joints generally require:

    A. no treatment, but transport to the hospital.

    B. immediate transport to the hospital by helicopter.

    C. slow, deliberate treatment and transport to the hospital.

    D. rapid treatment for life-threatening injury and transport to the hospital.

22. What is the longest, heaviest bone in the body?

    A. Tibia

    B. Ulna

    C. Femur

    D. Humerus

23. One of the fused joints in the adult body can be found at the:

    A. shoulder.

    B. cranium.

    C. elbow.

    D. knee.

24. The elbow is an example of a:

    A. ball-and-socket joint.

    B. joint capsule.

    C. hinge joint.

    D. trochanter.

106 Student Review Manual

The Musculoskeletal System

25. Which of the following bones consists of a body and a bony arch?

    A. Humerus

    B. Vertebra

    C. Femur

    D. Tibia

26. The sacrum and two pelvic bones comprise the pelvis. Each pelvic bone consists of how many parts?

    A. 1

    B. 3

    C. 5

    D. 7

27. The bones that make up the leg between the knee and the ankle are called the:

    A. tibia and the fibula.

    B. tibia and the radius.

    C. radius and the ulna.

    D. fibula and the ulna.

28. The bones that make up the forearm are called the:

    A. tibia and the fibula.

    B. tibia and the radius.

    C. radius and the ulna.

    D. fibula and the ulna.

29. How many pairs of ribs make up the rib cage?

    A. 8

    B. 10

    C. 12

    D. 14

Chapter 11

30. One of the functions of the skeletal system is to:

    A. serve as a reservoir for calcium, phosphorus, and other body chemicals.

    B. control the discharge of waste materials filtered from the blood.

    C. nourish and carry oxygen to different parts of the body.

    D. transmit messages between the brain and the body.

31. The human skeleton is made up of approximately how many bones?

    A. 150

    B. 200

    C. 250

    D. 300

32. The cartilaginous structure at the inferior end of the sternum is called the:

    A. scapula.

    B. clavicle.

    C. steroid process.

    D. xiphoid process.

33. Muscles can relax and contract, but they **CANNOT**:

    A. pull a bone.

    B. push a bone.

    C. aid in flexion.

    D. aid in extension.

34. A sprain usually occurs:

    A. at a joint.

    B. on the tuberosity.

    C. on the trochanter.

    D. along the shaft of the bone.

The Musculoskeletal System

35. The tough, connective tissues that attach bone to bone are called:

    A. tendrils.

    B. tendons.

    C. ligaments.

    D. mycocardia.

36. Which of the following bones forms the socket for a ball-and-socket joint?

    A. Patella

    B. Scapula

    C. Clavicle

    D. Sternum

37. The shoulder girdle is made up of the:

    A. clavicle, carpal, and phalanges.

    B. scapula, carpal, and metacarpals.

    C. scapula, carpal, and proximal humerus.

    D. scapula, clavicle, and proximal humerus.

38. The last two pairs of ribs are called floating ribs because they:

    A. connect directly to the sternum through a short bridge of cartilage.

    B. connect directly to the sternum through the costal arch.

    C. do not connect to the sternum or the thoracic vertebrae.

    D. do not connect to the sternum.

39. In addition to allowing body movement, skeletal muscles provide for:

    A. production of body heat.

    B. production of body cooling.

    C. transportation of oxygen.

    D. transportation of carbon dioxide.

Chapter 11

40. The type of muscle tissue found in the gastrointestinal tract is called:

   A. cardiac muscle.

   B. striated muscle.

   C. smooth muscle.

   D. voluntary muscle.

Answers

1:    **C.**   Voluntary, or skeletal, muscle allows bones to move. (ECTSI 5, p. 245)

2:    **B.**   The insertion of a muscle is on the distal point of the bone. (ECTSI 5, p. 246)

3:    **A.**   The tibia connects with the femur to form the knee joint. (ECTSI 5, p. 258)

4:    **C.**   The fifth through tenth ribs are those most commonly fractured. (ECTSI 5, p. 376)

5:    **B.**   The radius connects to the humerus. (ECTSI 5, p. 256)

6:    **C.**   The sternum joins the ribs at the front of the chest. (ECTSI 5, p. 254)

7:    **C.**   The maxilla and mandible make up the upper and lower aspects of the jaw. (ECTSI 5, p. 252)

8:    **A.**   A dislocation is the disruption of a joint. (ECTSI 5, p. 261)

9:    **B.**   The function of synovial fluid is to lubricate the bone ends at a joint. (ECTSI 5, p. 251)

10:    **D.**   Involuntary muscle carries out the automatic work of the body. (ECTSI 5, p. 246)

11:    **C.**   Electrical impulses carried from the brain and spinal cord along the peripheral nerves allow the skeletal muscle to contract. (ECTSI 5, pp. 245–246)

12:    **C.**   The biceps is composed of voluntary muscle. (ECTSI 5, p. 246)

The Musculoskeletal System

13: **D.** The diaphragm has characteristics of both voluntary and involuntary muscles. (ECTSI 5, p. 247)

14: **D.** Involuntary muscles are found in the walls of most tubular structures of the body, including the blood vessels. (ECTSI 5, p. 246)

15: **A.** The knee is a hinge joint. (ECTSI 5, p. 251)

16: **C.** Bone is the only tissue in the body that heals itself by forming more of itself. Other tissues in the body heal by forming scar tissue. (ECTSI 5, p. 249)

17: **A.** Of the options listed, the patella is most likely to dislocate. (ECTSI 5, pp. 255, 308)

18: **C.** The muscles lining the intestine wall are involuntary muscles. (ECTSI 5, p. 246)

19: **C.** Ball-and-socket joints allow motion in all directions. (ECTSI 5, p. 251)

20: **D.** Articular cartilage covers the ends of bones in joints where motion occurs. (ECTSI 5, pp. 250–251)

21: **C.** Patients with injuries to bones and joints generally require slow, deliberate treatment before being transported to the hospital. (ECTSI 5, p. 274)

22: **C.** The femur is the longest, heaviest bone in the body. (ECTSI 5, p. 257)

23: **B.** The cranium is one of the fused joints in the body. (ECTSI 5, pp. 249–250)

24: **C.** The elbow is an example of a hinge joint. (ECTSI 5, p. 256)

25: **B.** A vertebra consists of a solid block of bone in the front called the body and a bony arch in the back. (ECTSI 5, p. 253)

26: **B.** Each pelvic bone is formed by the fusion of three bones—the ilium, the ischium, and the pubis. (ECTSI 5, pp. 256–257)

27: **A.** The bones that make up the lower leg are called the tibia and the fibula. (ECTSI 5, pp. 258–259)

Chapter 11

28: **C.** The bones that make up the forearm are called the radius and the ulna. (ECTSI 5, p. 256)

29: **C.** Twelve pairs of ribs make up the rib cage. (ECTSI 5, p. 254)

30: **A.** One function of the skeletal system is to serve as a reservoir for calcium, phosphorus, and other body chemicals. (ECTSI 5, p. 247)

31: **B.** There are 206 bones in the skeleton. Of the options listed, 200 would be the correct answer. (ECTSI 5, p. 247)

32: **D.** The xiphoid process is one of three parts of the sternum. It is the cartilaginous structure located at the inferior end. (ECTSI 5, p. 254)

33: **B.** Muscles can relax and contract, but they cannot push a bone. (ECTSI 5, pp. 245–246)

34: **A.** A sprain usually occurs at a joint, dislocating it temporarily and tearing or stretching some of the supporting ligaments. (ECTSI 5, p. 261)

35: **C.** Ligaments are the tough, connective tissues that attach bone to bone. (ECTSI 5, p. 251)

36: **B.** The glenoid fossa, a region of the scapula, is the recess for the articulation of the humeral head. (ECTSI 5, p. 255)

37: **D.** The shoulder girdle is composed of the clavicle, scapula, and proximal humerus. (ECTSI 5, p. 255)

38: **D.** The last two pairs of ribs, the eleventh and twelfth ribs, are called floating ribs because they do not connect to the sternum. (ECTSI 5, p. 255)

39: **A.** Skeletal muscles produce body heat, which is released by the chemical reactions that cause skeletal muscles to contract. (ECTSI 5, p. 245)

40: **C.** Smooth muscle tissue lines the walls of the gastrointestinal tract. (ECTSI 5, p. 246)

Chapter 12

Fractures and Dislocations

Chapter Goals

The exercises in this chapter are designed to help the student to:

- identify various types of musculoskeletal injuries.

- list and describe various types of splints.

- describe how to assess various types of musculoskeletal injuries.

- describe how to apply various types of splints.

- explain how a traction splint differs from other splints.

- list the types of injuries for which a traction splint is needed.

Chapter 12

Multiple-Choice Questions

Select the correct answer for each of the following questions. Each question has only *one* correct or best answer.

1. A fractured elbow should be immobilized in the position in which it is found because movement may result in:

    A. further fracture.

    B. radial fracture.

    C. a dislocation.

    D. damage to nerves and blood vessels.

2. Which of the following statements about fractures is the most accurate?

    A. Fractures present no immediate threat to life.

    B. Few fractures present an immediate threat to life.

    C. Many fractures present an immediate threat to life.

    D. All fractures present an immediate threat to life.

3. An air splint should be inflated to the point in which:

    A. the wrinkles in the splint are about to disappear.

    B. the wrinkles in the splint have just disappeared.

    C. you can slightly dent the splint with thumb pressure.

    D. you cannot dent the splint with thumb pressure.

4. Of the following, which splint should **NOT** be used for an open fracture in which bone ends or fragments are protruding?

    A. Padded wooden board

    B. Padded wire or ladder splint

    C. Air splint

    D. Cardboard splint

Fractures and Dislocations

5. An injury in which ligaments are stretched or torn, usually from motion forcing them beyond the normal range of the joint, is called a:

    A. fracture.

    B. dislocation.

    C. sprain.

    D. strain.

6. When splinting an open fracture, you should:

    A. apply the splint before dressing the wound.

    B. dress the wound before applying the splint.

    C. allow the material that secures the splint to serve as the dressing.

    D. avoid dressing the wound, except in very minor compound fractures.

7. Of the following, which is the most reliable sign of a closed fracture?

    A. Visible bone fragment

    B. Point tenderness

    C. Swelling

    D. Bruising

8. Which of the following types of fractures is most commonly found in children?

    A. Greenstick

    B. Open

    C. Oblique

    D. Spiral

9. A patient with a fractured clavicle will typically sit or stand with the shoulder of the:

    A. injured side bent backward.

    B. injured side bent forward.

    C. uninjured side bent forward.

    D. uninjured side bent backward.

Chapter 12

10. The first step in assessing tenderness over the pelvis in a patient believed to have a pelvic fracture is to:

    A. gently move the knees toward the chest.

    B. press down on the symphysis pubis with the palm of your hand.

    C. place your hands over the lateral aspect of the iliac crests and compress.

    D. place your hands on top of the pelvic area and gently rock the pelvis side to side.

11. A patient has a "silver fork deformity" after falling on her outstretched hand. Immobilization should extend from the middle of the hand up to and including the:

    A. wrist.

    B. middle of the forearm.

    C. elbow.

    D. shoulder.

12. A 17-year-old boy dislocates his shoulder in a game of touch football. The patient is in extreme pain and shouts for you to "do something." Your first step in caring for the patient should be to:

    A. give him pain medication.

    B. give him supplemental oxygen.

    C. immobilize the shoulder in the position you found it.

    D. attempt to reduce or "put back in place" the shoulder.

13. A patient who is lying on the ground with his left leg bent out to the side appears to have a dislocated knee. He is in extreme pain and states that he cannot move the leg. On assessment, you find that the patient has strong distal pulses. You should prepare the patient for transport by:

    A. straightening the leg and applying two standard rigid leg splints.

    B. straightening the leg and applying and inflating an air splint.

    C. splinting the leg in the position in which it is found.

    D. wrapping the leg with a pillow.

Fractures and Dislocations

14. You should care for a patient with a suspected sprain:

    A. by applying cold compresses.

    B. by applying an elastic bandage.

    C. in the same manner as a patient with any minor injury.

    D. in the same manner as a patient with a fracture.

15. A dislocation is considered a high priority injury when there is:

    A. associated head injuries.

    B. severe swelling and bruising.

    C. severe angulation of the joint.

    D. loss of the distal pulse and/or sensation.

16. The best way to determine the location of a closed fracture in a conscious, alert patient is to:

    A. ask the patient where the pain is most severe.

    B. look for the area that is most swollen.

    C. feel the bone you believe is broken.

    D. look for areas of bruising.

17. When caring for a patient with a suspected extremity fracture, you should:

    A. move the limb to determine the severity of the fracture.

    B. move the limb across the body to provide support.

    C. splint the part in the position you find it, whenever possible.

    D. splint the part first, then control bleeding in open fractures.

Chapter 12

18. The principal purpose of splinting a fracture is to:

    A. reduce the fracture, if possible.

    B. force the bony fragments back into anatomic alignment.

    C. prevent motion of bony fragments.

    D. immobilize only the most serious fractures.

19. A fracture of the humeral shaft is most commonly immobilized with which of the following devices?

    A. Air splint

    B. Sager traction splint

    C. Padded wire ladder or Sam splint

    D. Padded board splint with a sling and swathe

20. A severely angulated fracture is considered serious because the angulation is likely to:

    A. pinch or cut nerves and blood vessels.

    B. cause the patient severe pain.

    C. make transport of the patient difficult.

    D. result in shortening of the limb.

21. A splint is applied to a patient with a fractured elbow. Five minutes later, the radial pulse in the injured arm is very weak, and the patient states that he has no feeling in the arm. Because the nearest hospital is 30 minutes away, the appropriate course of action would be to:

    A. transport the patient immediately.

    B. remove the splint, reposition the arm, and then reapply the splint.

    C. position the splinted arm lower than the patient's body.

    D. position the splinted arm higher than the patient's body.

Fractures and Dislocations

22. When splinting a fractured hand, you should be sure that the hand is:

    A. covered by the splint on the sides only.

    B. maintained in the position of function.

    C. splinted loose enough to allow some mobility.

    D. splinted to the shoulder.

23. The greatest danger associated with caring for a patient with a closed fracture is the possibility of which of the following complications?

    A. Hemorrhage

    B. Infection

    C. Shock

    D. Opening of the fracture

24. To effectively immobilize a fractured clavicle, you should apply:

    A. a sling and swathe.

    B. an air splint over the entire arm.

    C. a traction splint to the arm of the injured side.

    D. a rigid splint to the upper arm, then a sling.

25. A fractured patella is a common result of an automobile accident due to the impact of the:

    A. face against the steering wheel.

    B. knee against the dashboard.

    C. elbow against the dashboard.

    D. face and chest against the windshield.

Chapter 12

26. Sprains are injuries in which the:

    A. joint is dislocated.

    B. joint is fractured and the ligaments torn.

    C. ligaments around the joint are stretched or torn.

    D. muscles around the joints are stretched or torn.

27. Which of the following assessments requires that the patient be alert and cooperative?

    A. Monitoring the distal pulses

    B. Monitoring capillary refill

    C. Assessing sensation and motor function

    D. Assessing false motion

28. A patient who has a dislocated shoulder is found lying on her back. The patient should be transported to the hospital with the arm:

    A. straightened and splinted.

    B. placed in a sling and swathe.

    C. splinted in the position found.

    D. hanging of its own weight off the stretcher.

29. Which of the following assessment findings is **LEAST** likely to be associated with a severely angulated fracture of the humeral shaft?

    A. Wristdrop

    B. Numbness in the elbow

    C. Tingling sensations along the forearm

    D. Discoloration in the wrist and hand

Fractures and Dislocations

30. A woman appears to have fractures of the left leg and arm as a result of a head-on collision. The patient is conscious and states that her "stomach hurts." During your assessment, you notice a bloody discharge from the urethral area. You should prepare the patient for transport by immobilizing her on a:

    A. long spine board.

    B. long spine board with a PASG in place.

    C. stretcher, with her leg and arm supported with pillows.

    D. stretcher, with her leg in a traction splint and her arm in a sling.

31. An elderly patient who has a "hip fracture" as a result of a fall should be immobilized on a long spine board or scoop stretcher with the injured limb:

    A. gently realigned into proper anatomic position.

    B. supported with pillows in the position in which it was found.

    C. splinted with padded board splints from the hip to the ankle.

    D. secured in a traction splint.

32. After an extremity fracture is splinted, you should continually monitor the pulses:

    A. at the site of the injury.

    B. distal to the site of the injury.

    C. proximal to the site of the injury.

    D. in the uninjured limb only.

33. After grasping the limb above and below the fracture site, you should:

    A. slip the splint onto the site.

    B. apply steady traction as you apply the splint.

    C. push back exposed bone ends as you apply the splint.

    D. pull on the bone ends as you apply the splint.

Chapter 12

34. A 53-year-old man leaps from a third floor apartment window to escape a fire. The man tumbles in midair, but manages to land on his feet. The most appropriate course of action is to first:

    A. assess the patient thoroughly for third-degree burns.

    B. ask the man to come over to the ambulance immediately so he can be examined.

    C. treat any serious cuts and burns, then transport the patient to the hospital.

    D. treat the patient for impacted lower extremity fractures and possible fracture of the spine.

35. Proper immobilization of a fractured knee would include the:

    A. knee and femur only.

    B. knee, tibia, and fibula.

    C. ankle, tibia, fibula, and femur.

    D. ankle, tibia, fibula, femur, and hip.

36. Treatment of a suspected extremity fracture should include:

    A. elevating the limb above the level of the heart.

    B. splinting the injured bone, along with the joints above and below it.

    C. realigning the limb into normal anatomic alignment.

    D. moving the limb to determine the extent and severity of the fracture.

37. The best way to splint a fractured foot is with:

    A. a pillow.

    B. a sling and swathe.

    C. a ladder splint.

    D. a traction splint.

Fractures and Dislocations

38. The best way to splint a fractured rib is to:

    A. apply tape firmly around the entire chest.

    B. place the patient's arm over the fracture site and secure the arm with a sling and swathe.

    C. place a short wooden or cardboard splint over the fracture site and secure it with a sling and swathe.

    D. bend a ladder splint to the contour of the chest and secure it with tape.

39. Fractures of the femur are typically immobilized with:

    A. a ladder splint.

    B. a traction splint.

    C. an air splint.

    D. a long spine board.

40. The first step in applying a bishafted traction splint on a patient with a lower extremity fracture is to:

    A. ask your partner for assistance in applying the splint.

    B. slide the splint under the patient's leg.

    C. place the patient and the splint on a long spine board.

    D. connect the ankle hitch to the end of the splint.

41. Which of the following devices is **NOT** appropriate for use as an ankle hitch?

    A. Nylon strap with no shoe or sock

    B. Leather strap with no shoe or sock

    C. Web strap with no shoe or sock

    D. Adhesive tape with no shoe or sock

Chapter 12

42. Traction splints should not be used on upper extremity fractures because the countertraction forces of traction are:

    A. likely to exert too much pressure on the heart.

    B. too strong for the weaker bones in the upper extremity.

    C. too strong for the blood vessels and nerves in the axilla.

    D. ineffective with small splints, such as those needed for upper extremity fractures.

43. Proper immobilization of a fracture of the femur should include the:

    A. pelvis, hip, knee, and lower leg.

    B. hip, knee, and lower leg only.

    C. knee and lower leg only.

    D. lower leg only.

44. Which of the following statements about caring for a patient who has a closed fracture of the femur is true?

    A. Supplemental oxygen is of little value.

    B. Direct pressure will control the bleeding.

    C. A tourniquet should be applied above the fracture site.

    D. The patient should be monitored for signs and symptoms of shock.

45. A hip fracture has a characteristic appearance in which the injured leg is:

    A. rotated inward and apparently shortened.

    B. rotated inward, but not shortened.

    C. rotated outward and apparently shortened.

    D. angled backward, but not shortened.

Fractures and Dislocations

46. When applying a traction splint, you should apply longitudinal pull until the:

    A. limb has straightened completely.

    B. limb sufficiently fits into the splint.

    C. bone ends realign.

    D. fracture is reduced.

47. A patient believed to have a fractured femur should be splinted appropriately and also treated for possible:

    A. shock.

    B. anaphylaxis.

    C. cardiovascular accident.

    D. myocardial infarction.

48. Which of the following devices should **NOT** be used for a patient who has a hip fracture?

    A. Long spine board

    B. Traction splint

    C. Split litter

    D. Air splint

49. Of the following, which is the most important reason for using a traction splint?

    A. To reduce a fracture

    B. To realign bone ends

    C. To stabilize a broken bone

    D. To stretch a broken limb until the broken ends slip back into place

Chapter 12

Answers

1: **D.** A fractured elbow should be immobilized in the position in which it is found because movement may result in damage to nerves and blood vessels. (ECTSI 5, p. 293)

2: **B.** Few fractures present an immediate threat to life. (ECTSI 5, p. 282)

3: **C.** An air splint should be inflated to the point in which you can slightly dent the splint with thumb pressure. (ECTSI 5, p. 277)

4: **C.** An air splint should not be used when bone ends are protruding since the pressure of the splint could force the bone ends into the skin or puncture the splint. (ECTSI 5, p. 193)

5: **C.** A sprain results when ligaments are stretched or torn. (ECTSI 5, p. 261)

6: **B.** When splinting an open fracture, you should dress the wound before applying the splint. (ECTSI 5, p. 275)

7: **B.** While all of the signs listed occur with closed fractures, the most reliable sign of underlying fracture is point tenderness. (ECTSI 5, p. 268)

8: **A.** Greenstick fractures are most commonly found in infants and children. (ECTSI 5, p. 267)

9: **B.** A patient with a fractured clavicle will typically sit or stand with the shoulder of the injured side bent forward. (ECTSI 5, pp. 285–286)

10: **C.** Assessment for a possible fracture of the pelvis should begin by placing your hands over the lateral aspect of the iliac crests and then compressing the pelvic ring. Then place your palms over the anterior aspect of the iliac crests and apply firm downward pressure. Palpate the symphysis pubis last. (ECTSI 5, pp. 300–301)

11: **C.** Immobilization of a Colles' fracture, or "silver fork deformity," should extend from the middle of the hand up to and including the elbow joint. You may also add a sling or supporting pillow to make the patient more comfortable. (ECTSI 5, pp. 294–295)

12: **C.** A patient with a dislocated shoulder will be in extreme pain; therefore, immobilization is difficult. You should immobilize the shoulder in the position in which you found it to avoid producing more pain. Never attempt to reduce or "put back in place" the shoulder. (ECTSI 5, p. 289)

Fractures and Dislocations

13: **C.** A patient with a dislocated knee will be in extreme pain. If the patient has strong distal pulses in the injured leg, splint the knee in the position in which you found it. (ECTSI 5, p. 307)

14: **D.** Without X rays, it is impossible to rule out a fracture; therefore, a patient with a suspected strain or sprain should be treated in the same manner as a patient believed to have a fracture. (ECTSI 5, p. 270)

15: **D.** A dislocation is considered a high priority injury when there is loss of the distal pulse or loss of sensation. (ECTSI 5, p. 307)

16: **A.** In a conscious, alert patient, the best way to determine the location of a closed fracture is to ask the patient where the pain is most severe. (ECTSI 5, p. 268)

17: **C.** You should splint a suspected extremity fracture in the position in which you found it whenever possible. (ECTSI 5, p. 275)

18: **C.** The principal purpose of splinting a fracture is to prevent motion of the bony fragments. Basic splinting is not meant to force fragments into anatomic alignment, nor is it reserved for only "serious fractures." You should never try to reduce a fracture. (ECTSI 5, pp. 274–275)

19: **D.** A fracture of the humeral shaft is most commonly splinted with a padded board splint. (ECTSI 5, p. 290)

20: **A.** Angulation may cause pinching or cutting of nerves and blood vessels. (ECTSI 5, p. 290)

21: **B.** The appropriate course of action in this situation would be one attempt to remove the splint, reposition the arm, and then reapply the splint. (ECTSI 5, p. 294)

22: **B.** The hand should always be maintained in the position of function by having the patient grasp a roll of gauze. (ECTSI 5, p. 296)

23: **D.** The greatest danger is the possibility of causing the fracture to open, or become compound, by mishandling it. (ECTSI 5, p. 274)

24: **A.** A sling and swathe is used to immobilize a fractured clavicle. (ECTSI 5, pp. 286–287)

25: **B.** Fractures of the patella are often caused by a knee impacting against the dashboard. (ECTSI 5, p. 265)

Chapter 12

26: **C.** Sprains occur when the ligaments around the joints are stretched or torn. (ECTSI 5, p. 261)

27: **C.** Assessments of sensation and motor function require that the patient be alert and cooperative. (ECTSI 5, p. 272)

28: **C.** In this situation, splint and then immobilize the shoulder in the position you found it in before you transport the patient to the hospital. (ECTSI 5, p. 289)

29: **D.** A patient who has a severely angulated fracture of the humeral shaft should be assessed for the characteristic wristdrop that occurs when the radial nerve is compressed, lacerated, or trapped at the fracture site. Numbness and tingling are also common with this type of fracture. (ECTSI 5, p. 290)

30: **B.** The patient's abdominal pain and bloody discharge suggest a possible pelvic fracture. The appropriate course of action in this situation would be to immobilize the patient on a long spine board with a PASG in place under the patient. (ECTSI 5, p. 300)

31: **B.** An elderly patient who sustains a hip fracture as a result of a fall should be placed on a long spine board or scoop stretcher with the injured limb supported with pillows or rolled blankets in the position in which you found it. (ECTSI 5, pp. 303–304)

32: **B.** After an extremity fracture is splinted, you should continually monitor the pulses distal to the site of injury to determine if the splint has impaired circulation to the rest of the limb. (ECTSI 5, pp. 275–278)

33: **B.** As you prepare to apply a splint, grasp the limb above and below the fracture site, then apply steady traction as you apply the splint. (ECTSI 5, pp. 275–277)

34: **D.** In this situation, you should suspect impacted fractures of the lower extremities and possible fractures of the spine. (ECTSI 5, p. 310)

35: **D.** The entire extremity, including the hip, should be immobilized. (ECTSI 5, pp. 307–308)

36: **B.** Treatment of a suspected extremity fracture should include splinting the bone and joints above and below the fracture site. If the joint is injured, you should splint the joint and the bones adjacent to it. (ECTSI 5, p. 275)

Fractures and Dislocations

37: **A.** Of the choices given, the best way to splint a fractured foot is with a pillow. The pillow will splint the foot and protect it without causing undue pressure. (ECTSI 5, p. 311)

38: **B.** The best way to splint a fractured rib is to place the patient's arm over the fracture site and secure the arm with a sling and swathe. (ECTSI 5, p. 375)

39: **B.** Unless contraindicated, fractures of the femur are typically immobilized with a traction splint. (ECTSI 5, p. 304)

40: **A.** The first step in applying a bishafted traction splint on a patient with a lower extremity fracture is to ask your partner for assistance in applying the splint. This type of traction splint, such as the Hare Traction Splint, requires at least two operators. (ECTSI 5, pp. 280–281)

41: **D.** Adhesive tape should not be used as an ankle hitch because the tape should not be applied directly on the skin. (ECTSI 5, p. 282)

42: **C.** Traction splints should not be used on upper extremity fractures because the countertraction forces of traction are too strong for the blood vessels and nerves in the axilla. (ECTSI 5, pp. 279–280)

43: **A.** The pelvis, hip, knee, and lower leg should all be immobilized in this situation. (ECTSI 5, pp. 280–281, 305)

44: **D.** A patient with a closed fracture of the femur should be monitored for signs and symptoms of shock. The patient could lose enough blood into the soft tissues to go into shock. (ECTSI 5, p. 304)

45: **C.** A hip fracture has a characteristic appearance in which the injured leg is rotated outward and apparently shortened. (ECTSI 5, p. 303)

46: **B.** When applying a traction splint, you should apply longitudinal pull to align the limb sufficiently to fit into the splint. (ECTSI 5, p. 275)

47: **A.** A patient with a fractured femur should also be treated for shock. (ECTSI 5, p. 304)

48: **D.** An air splint will not immobilize a hip fracture. (ECTSI 5, p. 277)

49: **C.** The most important reason to use a traction splint is to stabilize a broken bone. (ECTSI 5, p. 275)

Chapter 13

Spinal Injuries

Chapter Goals

The exercises in this chapter are designed to help the student to:

- identify the parts of the spine.

- describe common injuries to the spine.

- identify common signs and symptoms of spinal injury.

- explain basic principles of immobilization.

- describe appropriate use of several devices used for immobilization.

- list common complications of spinal injury.

Spinal Injuries

Multiple-Choice Questions

Select the correct answer for each of the following questions. Each question has only *one* correct or best answer.

1. The sacral spine contains how many vertebrae?

    A. 4

    B. 5

    C. 7

    D. 12

2. The vertebrae of the sacral spine are unique in that they are:

    A. fused.

    B. gliding joints.

    C. hinge joints.

    D. ball-and-socket joints.

3. The spinal column is made up of 33 bones and is divided into how many sections?

    A. 3

    B. 4

    C. 5

    D. 6

4. The first seven vertebrae of the spinal column are referred to as the:

    A. sacral spine.

    B. cervical spine.

    C. lumbar spine.

    D. thoracic spine.

Chapter 13

5. What parts of the spinal column are most commonly injured?

   A. Cervical and thoracic

   B. Cervical and lumbar

   C. Cervical and sacral

   D. Lumbar and thoracic

6. Obvious deformity of the spine is rare, but when it does occur, it is most often seen with an injury to the:

   A. sacrum.

   B. lumbar spine.

   C. cervical spine.

   D. thoracic spine.

7. Assessment of a patient who has an injury of the cervical spine is most likely to show paralysis of the:

   A. facial and chest muscles.

   B. neck and rupture of the diaphragm.

   C. chest muscles and respiratory difficulty.

   D. chest muscles and rupture of the diaphragm.

8. A man is found slumped over the steering wheel, unconscious and making "snoring" sounds, after an automobile accident. The patient's head is turned to the side, and his neck is flexed. The first step in caring for this patient would be to carefully:

   A. splint the head in the position you found it.

   B. rotate the head to correct the deformity.

   C. hyperextend the neck to correct the deformity.

   D. attempt manual stabilization and move the head to a neutral, in-line position.

Spinal Injuries

9. A patient with suspected spinal injuries should be immobilized on a short backboard during extrication and then:

    A. secured onto the ambulance stretcher.

    B. secured onto a full backboard.

    C. fitted with foam head blocks.

    D. fitted with a cervical collar, followed by placement onto the ambulance stretcher.

10. A woman found sitting in her car after an automobile accident is believed to have a spinal injury. The most appropriate short-term immobilization device would be a cervical collar, along with a:

    A. long backboard.

    B. short backboard.

    C. semirigid litter.

    D. pneumatic antishock garment (PASG).

11. The lumbar spine consists of how many vertebrae?

    A. 4

    B. 5

    C. 7

    D. 12

12. What part of the spinal column is often injured as a result of lifting a heavy object improperly?

    A. Cervical

    B. Thoracic

    C. Lumbar

    D. Sacral

Chapter 13

13. The principal function of an intervertebral disc is to:

    A. carry blood to the vertebrae.

    B. provide for nerve function in the vertebrae.

    C. control motion of and between the vertebrae.

    D. serve as a point of attachment between the spinal cord and muscles in the back.

14. Which of the following areas of the spine is supported by other bones in the thorax?

    A. Lumbar

    B. Thoracic

    C. Sacrum

    D. Coccyx

15. What is the minimum number of EMTs needed to properly logroll a patient who has a cervical spine injury?

    A. 3

    B. 4

    C. 5

    D. 6

16. A man is found unconscious, slumped over the steering wheel, after an automobile accident. He regains consciousness and is able to feel pain in his hands and feet. This finding suggests that the:

    A. patient has a hematoma.

    B. cervical spine has been displaced.

    C. back has not been seriously injured.

    D. spinal cord has not been cut or severed.

Spinal Injuries

17. Assessing for spinal injuries is made easier if the patient is:

    A. conscious and on his or her back.

    B. conscious and on his or her side.

    C. unconscious and on his or her back.

    D. unconscious and on his or her side.

18. A woman has chest and abdominal injuries as a result of a head-on collision in which she was driving about 40 mph. The patient was not wearing a seat belt, but states that she has no head or back pain. Her injuries suggest that she hit the steering wheel on impact. The appropriate course of action would be to:

    A. treat the chest and abdominal wounds first, without concern about possible spinal injuries.

    B. treat for possible spinal injuries first, then concentrate on her other injuries.

    C. treat for possible spinal injuries only; the possibility of a severed spinal cord makes the other injuries less important.

    D. contact medical control to establish priorities of care.

19. A 17-year-old boy is found unconscious, floating facedown in a swimming pool. You and your partner should first:

    A. roll him over as a unit and then place him on a backboard.

    B. place him on a backboard in a facedown position, then remove him from the pool.

    C. stabilize his neck and back with your hands while you and your partner roll him over as a unit and then establish an open airway.

    D. roll him over as a unit, extend his neck to open the airway, and then prepare to float a backboard under him.

20. As a patient is being logrolled, one EMT should remain at the patient's head primarily to:

    A. keep the patient awake.

    B. monitor the straps and cravats.

    C. maintain manual cervical support.

    D. call out logrolling commands.

Chapter 13

21. The proper sequence for treating a patient with possible spinal injuries is to first complete the primary survey and then:

    A. establish an open airway.

    B. immobilize the entire body.

    C. apply and maintain manual cervical support.

    D. perform a thorough survey of the body.

22. A woman cannot move her arms or legs after an automobile accident. These findings suggest that the woman has injured her:

    A. peripheral nerves.

    B. spinal cord in the cervical region.

    C. spinal cord in the thoracic region.

    D. spinal cord in the sacral region.

23. You alone are the first to arrive at the scene of an automobile accident. A man is conscious, lying on his back on the ground next to his automobile. The patient cannot move his legs and states that his "back hurts." Your first step in caring for this patient would be to:

    A. roll him gently to his stomach and place a pillow under his head.

    B. gently raise him to a sitting position and ask if this relieves the pain.

    C. gently lift him onto a stretcher and transport him to the hospital.

    D. leave him on his back, tell him to remain still, and then call for backup.

24. A patient who has a spinal injury must be moved. As you begin to move the patient, you should make sure that the spinal column is:

    A. well padded.

    B. wrapped tightly.

    C. in traction.

    D. in a straight line.

Spinal Injuries

25. The thoracic spine is made up of how many vertebrae?

    A. 4

    B. 5

    C. 7

    D. 12

26. A 5-year-old child requires full spinal immobilization after falling from a tree. As the child is logrolled onto the backboard, you should:

    A. place a small pillow under the child's head to prevent hyperextension of the neck.

    B. place a rolled towel under the child's neck to prevent hyperextension of the neck.

    C. place blanket rolls under the child's knees to prevent the legs from moving.

    D. place padding between the shoulders and the backboard to prevent hyperflexion of the neck.

27. The windshield is broken on the passenger's side after an automobile accident. You would expect to first provide care for possible:

    A. eye injuries.

    B. facial injuries.

    C. cervical spine injuries.

    D. lumbar spine injuries.

28. An unconscious patient with possible spinal injuries seems to have trouble breathing. The patient's chest wall is moving only slightly, but the diaphragm is moving in and out with each breath. These findings suggest that the patient:

    A. needs CPR immediately.

    B. needs supplemental oxygen immediately, and possibly assisted ventilations.

    C. is breathing normally following trauma, but requires immediate transport.

    D. should be placed in Trendelenburg's position to increase blood flow to the heart.

Chapter 13

29. A man is conscious and alert after an automobile accident in which he was the driver. He states that his fingers are tingling and that his shoulders hurt. Your assessment should include:

    A. gently feeling along the spine for any point tenderness.

    B. gently moving the patient's arms, legs, and shoulders to determine the severity of his pain.

    C. asking the patient to roll and shrug his shoulders in an attempt to determine the severity of his pain.

    D. asking the patient to move his head from side to side to determine if he has neck pain.

30. Motor nerves conduct impulses from the:

    A. sensory fibers to the brain.

    B. brain to the sensory fibers.

    C. brain to the muscles.

    D. muscles to the brain.

31. The membranes surrounding the brain and spinal cord are called:

    A. pleurae.

    B. meninges.

    C. mesenteries.

    D. parietal pleura.

32. Which of the following statements about spinal cord injuries is true?

    A. All injuries to the spinal cord can be corrected with surgery.

    B. A severed spinal cord can be surgically repaired.

    C. A severed spinal cord can repair itself with proper immobilization.

    D. An injured spinal cord has limited self-healing abilities.

Spinal Injuries

33. A "whiplash" injury most commonly occurs to which of the following sections of the spine?

    A. Cervical

    B. Thoracic

    C. Lumbar

    D. Sacral

34. A woman with suspected spinal injuries as a result of an automobile accident must be removed from the vehicle. Your choice of immobilization device should be based primarily on:

    A. distance to the nearest hospital.

    B. your comfort level with various devices.

    C. position and condition of the patient only.

    D. position and condition of the patient, as well as type and condition of the vehicle.

Answers

1: **B.** The sacral spine in an adult consists of five fused vertebrae. (ECTSI 5, p. 253)

2: **A.** The vertebrae of the sacral spine are unique in that they are fused. (ECTSI 5, p. 253)

3: **C.** The 33 bones of the spinal column are divided into five sections. (ECTSI 5, p. 253)

4: **B.** The first seven vertebrae of the spinal column are referred to as the cervical spine. (ECTSI 5, p. 253)

5: **B.** The cervical and lumbar sections of the spine are most commonly injured. The thoracic section is protected by the shoulder girdle and ribs, and the sacrum is protected by the pelvic bones. (ECTSI 5, p. 253)

Chapter 13

6: **C.** While obvious deformity associated with spinal injury is rare, it may occur. When present, deformity is most commonly seen in cervical spine injuries. (ECTSI 5, p. 337)

7: **C.** Assessment of a patient with a cervical spine injury may reveal paralysis of the chest muscles, with resulting respiratory difficulty. (ECTSI 5, pp. 338, 348)

8: **D.** The patient's "snoring" sounds indicate an airway problem. Therefore, you should attempt manual stabilization and gently move the head to a neutral, in-line position. (ECTSI 5, p. 340)

9: **B.** A patient with possible spinal injuries should be immobilized on a short backboard during extrication, but then secured onto a long backboard prior to transport. The ambulance stretcher will not provide adequate immobilization, and the foam head blocks do not provide full immobilization. (ECTSI 5, p. 348)

10: **B.** The most appropriate short-term immobilization device for this patient is a cervical collar in conjunction with a short backboard. A long backboard should be used once the patient has been extricated from the vehicle. (ECTSI 5, pp. 346–348)

11: **B.** The lumbar spine consists of five vertebrae. (ECTSI 5, p. 253)

12: **C.** The lumbar spine is most likely to be injured as a result of improper lifting technique, due to bending at the waist and lower back. (ECTSI 5, p. 676)

13: **C.** The principal purpose of the intervertebral disc is to control motion of and between the vertebrae. The discs also protect the vertebrae from rubbing against each other. (ECTSI 5, p. 254)

14: **B.** The thoracic spine is supported by the ribs. (ECTSI 5, p. 253)

15: **B.** Ideally, four EMTs are needed to properly logroll a patient. (ECTSI 5, p. 684)

16: **D.** In this situation, you know that the spinal cord has not been severed because the patient feels pain in the extremities. However, you should assume that the patient has spinal injuries and provide care accordingly. (ECTSI 5, p. 337)

Spinal Injuries

17: **A.** Assessing for spinal injuries is much easier if the patient is conscious and lying on his or her back. A conscious patient is able to describe pain and various other symptoms. Assessment is less complicated if the patient is in a supine (on the back) position, as you do not need to move the patient to complete your assessment. (ECTSI 5, p. 339)

18: **B.** The most appropriate course of action in any situation in which spinal injuries are a possibility is to address the possible spinal injuries first, then concentrate on other injuries. (ECTSI 5, p. 338)

19: **C.** The first step in caring for a patient who is found unconscious, floating facedown in a pool, is for you and your partner to stabilize the patient's neck and back with your hands. You should then roll him over as a unit and establish an airway while you are still in the water. (ECTSI 5, p. 638)

20: **C.** As a patient is being logrolled, one EMT should remain at the patient's head in order to maintain manual cervical support. (ECTSI 5, p. 684)

21: **C.** As you complete the primary survey of a patient who has possible spinal injuries, you should apply and maintain manual cervical support. Establishing the airway is part of the primary survey. (ECTSI 5, p. 342)

22: **B.** A patient who cannot move his or her arms or legs after a high-velocity automobile accident has likely injured the cervical spine. (ECTSI 5, p. 338)

23: **D.** In this situation, especially when you are alone, you would leave the patient on his back, tell him to remain still, and then call for help. The patient has likely sustained spinal injuries and any movement should be avoided to prevent additional injury. (ECTSI 5, pp. 338–339)

24: **D.** As you prepare to move a patient with a spinal injury, you should make sure that the patient's airway is clear and that the spinal column is immobilized in a straight line. (ECTSI 5, pp. 342–343)

25: **D.** The thoracic spine is made up of 12 vertebrae. (ECTSI 5, p. 253)

26: **D.** As you logroll a child onto an immobilization device, make sure you place padding under the child's shoulders to prevent hyperflexion of the neck. (ECTSI 5, p. 344)

27: **C.** In any high-velocity accident, such as a collision in which the head hits the windshield, you should treat the patient for possible cervical spine injuries first, then concentrate on other injuries. (ECTSI 5, p. 337)

Chapter 13

28: **B.** An unconscious patient who is breathing with his diaphragm rather than with his chest muscles has likely sustained a severe spinal injury. When the diaphragm is unable to substitute for the chest muscles, the patient is likely to have respiratory difficulty. Therefore, you should give the patient supplemental oxygen at 100%, monitor breathing, and prepare to assist ventilations if necessary. (ECTSI 5, pp. 348–349)

29: **A.** A patient who is conscious and complaining of shoulder pain and tingling in the extremities should be treated for possible spinal injuries. Your assessment should include gently feeling along the spine for any point tenderness. You should not ask the patient to move the head, neck, or extremities to prevent further injury. (ECTSI 5, p. 337)

30: **C.** Motor nerves conduct impulses from the brain to the muscles. (ECTSI 5, p. 317)

31: **B.** The meninges are membranes that surround the brain and the spinal cord. (ECTSI 5, p. 320)

32: **D.** An injured spinal cord has only very limited self-healing abilities. A severed spinal cord cannot be repaired. Once damaged, cells in the brain and spinal cord cannot be reproduced or regenerated. (ECTSI 5, p. 320)

33: **A.** The cervical spine is most commonly affected when a whiplash injury occurs. (ECTSI 5, p. 337)

34: **D.** Your choice of immobilization device should be based on the patient's medical condition and the physical situation in which you find the patient, such as the condition of the vehicle. (ECTSI 5, p. 706)

Chapter 14

Injuries of the Head, Eyes, Mouth, and Face

Chapter Goals

The exercises in this chapter are designed to help the student to:

- describe the signs and symptoms of a head injury.

- explain why any bleeding within the skull is a serious medical condition.

- explain the importance of assessing level of consciousness associated with head injuries.

- describe the anatomy of the eye.

- explain why airway management is so important in the treatment of facial injuries.

- identify appropriate treatment of specific injuries of the head, eyes, mouth, and face.

Chapter 14

Multiple-Choice Questions

Select the correct answer for each of the following questions. Each question has only *one* correct or best answer.

1. The best way to control bleeding from the carotid artery is to apply:

    A. a tourniquet.

    B. pressure dressings.

    C. direct manual pressure.

    D. multitrauma dressings.

2. Cerebrospinal fluid leaking from the ear, nose, or scalp will most commonly appear as a:

    A. thick, clear fluid.

    B. thick, dark red fluid.

    C. watery, dark red fluid.

    D. watery, clear or pink fluid.

3. The circular muscle behind the cornea that regulates the amount of light entering the eye is called the:

    A. iris.

    B. lens.

    C. sclera.

    D. retina.

4. The globe-like shape of the eye is maintained by the:

    A. iris.

    B. retina.

    C. vitreous humor.

    D. muscles and ligaments.

Injuries of the Head, Eyes, Mouth, and Face

5. A patient with a serious head injury is most likely to have a:

   A. higher than normal blood pressure and slower than normal pulse.

   B. lower than normal blood pressure and slower than normal pulse.

   C. higher than normal blood pressure and faster than normal pulse.

   D. lower than normal blood pressure and faster than normal pulse.

6. The first step in caring for a patient with a severe facial injury is to:

   A. ensure that the airway is clear.

   B. check for bleeding inside the mouth.

   C. apply direct pressure with a dry, sterile dressing.

   D. stabilize the cervical spine.

7. The clear structure of the eye in front of the iris is called the:

   A. lens.

   B. sclera.

   C. retina.

   D. cornea.

8. The most serious underlying problem associated with a facial injury is:

   A. fracture of facial bones.

   B. injury to the lumbar spine.

   C. partial or complete upper airway obstruction.

   D. possible hypovolemic shock.

9. Treatment of a patient with forehead lacerations and a possible depressed skull fracture should include:

   A. applying a bandage using firm pressure to stop the bleeding.

   B. leaving the wound open to avoid putting pressure on the fracture.

   C. applying a dry, sterile dressing and elevating the patient's head slightly.

   D. applying a dry, sterile dressing and lowering the patient's head slightly.

Chapter 14

10. Bleeding from the ears and dark discoloration under the eyes following traumatic injuries suggest a:

    A. concussion.

    B. fractured skull.

    C. cerebral thrombosis.

    D. cerebrovascular accident.

11. The first step in treating a patient with a head injury is to:

    A. control bleeding.

    B. immobilize the patient's head.

    C. establish and maintain an airway.

    D. check for and stabilize any cervical spine injuries.

12. A foreign object impaled in the globe of the eye should be managed by:

    A. placing a loose dressing over the object and bandaging the injured eye.

    B. removing the object from the eye, closing the eyelid, and bandaging both eyes with pressure dressings.

    C. applying a doughnut dressing around the object, securing it with gauze dressing, and patching the uninjured eye.

    D. applying a doughnut dressing around the object, securing it with gauze dressing, and leaving the uninjured eye unbandaged.

13. Fracture of the larynx is most likely to occur in any crushing injury of the:

    A. face.

    B. neck.

    C. clavicle.

    D. sternum.

146 Student Review Manual

Injuries of the Head, Eyes, Mouth, and Face

14. A portion of a patient's ear is completely avulsed as a result of a fight. You should attempt to find the avulsed part and then:

    A. dispose of it so the patient does not become upset.

    B. reposition it on the injury site with sterile dressings and tape.

    C. place it in a container of cool water and transport it with the patient.

    D. place it in a moist, sterile dressing in a plastic bag inside a cool container, and transport it with the patient.

15. When treating a patient with an injury to one eye, you should cover both eyes to reduce:

    A. fear and anxiety.

    B. collateral circulation.

    C. sympathetic movement.

    D. tearing and paradoxical movement.

16. Which of the following acts as a shock absorber for the brain and spinal cord?

    A. The skull

    B. The dura mater

    C. The blood vessels

    D. The cerebrospinal fluid

17. Irrigation with water or sterile saline solution is the treatment of choice for what type of eye injury?

    A. Laceration

    B. Thermal burn

    C. Chemical burn

    D. A small foreign body embedded in the eye

Chapter 14

18. The first step in maintaining the airway of an unconscious patient with a head injury is to:

    A. sweep the mouth clear.

    B. hyperextend the jaw and cervical spine.

    C. extend the neck with the head-tilt maneuver.

    D. stabilize the head and cervical spine in a neutral, in-line position.

19. The first step in emergency treatment for a child who sprayed oven cleaner in his eyes is to:

    A. provide immediate transport to the hospital.

    B. provide continuous irrigation en route to the hospital.

    C. call the poison control center and then bandage the eyes.

    D. neutralize the chemical with lemon juice or vinegar and then provide transport to the hospital.

20. If cerebrospinal fluid is present in the ear or nose after a head injury, you should:

    A. pack the ears and nose.

    B. cover the ears and nose loosely.

    C. cover the ears and nose tightly.

    D. pack the ears, but allow the nose to drain.

21. An unconscious patient with a head injury may have brain damage if the pupils of the eyes are:

    A. unequal.

    B. constricted.

    C. paradoxical.

    D. equal and reactive.

Injuries of the Head, Eyes, Mouth, and Face

22. A sliver of glass penetrates through a patient's cheek into the mouth. You should attempt to:

    A. remove the glass and irrigate the wound with sterile water or saline solution.

    B. remove the glass and hold gauze against both the inside and outside of the cheek.

    C. leave the glass in place and hold gauze against both the inside and outside of the cheek.

    D. tilt the patient's head to the uninjured side and slightly lower the cheek and mouth without flexing the neck.

23. An adult patient with a head injury goes into shock. You should suspect:

    A. concussion.

    B. brain damage.

    C. cerebral edema.

    D. another serious injury.

24. During a self-defense class, a 20-year-old man falls to the ground after he is struck in the throat by his partner's fist. You should first determine if:

    A. the trachea is fractured.

    B. there is a patent airway.

    C. there is a strong carotid pulse.

    D. air is escaping into the soft tissue of the neck.

25. A patient who is unconscious immediately after an automobile accident, regains consciousness upon your arrival. You should suspect a:

    A. stroke.

    B. fainting episode.

    C. skull fracture.

    D. closed head injury.

Chapter 14

26. The function of the meninges is to:

    A. protect the heart.

    B. surround the lungs.

    C. surround and protect the brain and spinal cord.

    D. connect the intestines to the abdominal wall.

27. The spinal cord is considered:

    A. a continuation of the brainstem.

    B. a separate organ, detached from the brain.

    C. an independent organ, connected to the brain by muscle.

    D. an independent organ, attached to the brain by vertebrae.

28. The dura mater is a protective covering for the:

    A. brain.

    B. lungs.

    C. larynx.

    D. abdomen.

29. A woman hits her head on a low tree branch while she is riding a moped. You find her lying on the sidewalk with a large abrasion over her left eye. Her partner states that the patient seemed fine after she ran into the tree, but about 5 minutes later she did not remember where she was or what she was doing. The patient is alert now, but agitated. The most appropriate course of action would be to:

    A. bandage her abrasion and take her home, since she is now alert.

    B. bandage her abrasion, and send her home with instructions to call her personal physician.

    C. monitor her for further changes in level of consciousness during transport.

    D. monitor her for further changes in level of consciousness and if there are none, send her home.

Injuries of the Head, Eyes, Mouth, and Face

30. Because the face and scalp are well supplied with arteries and veins, they are said to be:

    A. cervical.

    B. vascular.

    C. muscular.

    D. epidermal.

31. The first step in treating a bleeding head wound should consist of:

    A. applying pressure to the subclavian artery.

    B. lightly packing the wound with sterile dressings.

    C. applying local manual pressure with a dry, sterile dressing.

    D. applying a loose, sterile dressing to aid the clotting process.

32. A patient has a small metal rod impaled in the skull. You should:

    A. remove the rod and apply a loose, sterile dressing.

    B. leave the rod in place and stabilize it with dressings.

    C. remove the rod and pack the wound with sterile pads.

    D. leave the rod in place unless it will hinder transport of the patient.

33. Because of possible airway difficulties, an unconscious patient with facial injuries should be properly immobilized and transported in a:

    A. side-lying position.

    B. supine position.

    C. sitting position, with the head tilted backward.

    D. sitting position, with the head between the legs.

Chapter 14

34. Permanent loss of vision may be prevented in a patient who has a lacerated eyelid, as long as there is no damage to the:

    A. globe.

    B. conjunctiva.

    C. lacrimal duct.

    D. superior lacrimal gland.

35. Swelling of the brain after injury is considered serious, because:

    A. swelling may travel to the spinal cord.

    B. it is difficult to drain fluid from the skull.

    C. pressure on the brain may cause a hemorrhage.

    D. there is little room for expansion within the skull.

36. Fractures of the facial bones are considered serious, because:

    A. associated bleeding is not easily stopped.

    B. they generally cause permanent scarring.

    C. they are not easily repaired without surgery.

    D. the patient is at risk for possible airway obstruction.

37. Discoloration of the soft tissues around the eye as a result of a head injury is called:

    A. ecchymosis.

    B. Battle's sign.

    C. cerebral edema.

    D. epidural hematoma.

38. The AVPU scale provides a baseline evaluation of a patient's:

    A. mental status.

    B. visual acuity.

    C. response to pain.

    D. level of consciousness.

Injuries of the Head, Eyes, Mouth, and Face

39. Supplemental oxygen should always be given routinely to a patient who has a head injury to minimize what two problems?

    A. Amnesia and dizziness

    B. Cyanosis and vomiting blood

    C. Confusion and dizziness

    D. Brain swelling and hypoxia

Answers

1: **C.** Applying direct manual pressure is the best way to control bleeding from the carotid artery. (ECTSI 5, pp. 367–368)

2: **D.** Cerebrospinal fluid leaking from the ear, nose, or scalp appears as a watery, clear or pink fluid. (ECTSI 5, p. 326)

3: **A.** The iris is the circular muscle that regulates the amount of light entering the eye. (ECTSI 5, p. 352)

4: **C.** The vitreous humor gives the eye its globe-like shape. (ECTSI 5, p. 351)

5: **A.** Higher than normal blood pressure and slower than normal pulse suggest that a patient has a serious head injury. (ECTSI 5, p. 329)

6: **A.** The first step in caring for a patient with a severe facial injury is to ensure that the airway is clear. (ECTSI 5, p. 363)

7: **D.** The cornea is the clear structure in front of the iris. (ECTSI 5, p. 351)

8: **C.** The most serious underlying problem associated with a facial injury is partial or complete upper airway obstruction. (ECTSI 5, p. 363)

9: **C.** Treatment of forehead lacerations and a possible depressed skull fracture includes applying a dry, sterile dressing, without applying pressure, and then elevating the patient's head slightly. (ECTSI 5, pp. 330–332)

10: **B.** Bleeding from the ears and dark discoloration under the eyes are indicators of a fractured skull. (ECTSI 5, p. 324)

11: **C.** Establishing and maintaining an airway is the first step in treating a patient with a head injury. (ECTSI 5, p. 328)

Chapter 14

12: **C.** A foreign object impaled in the globe of the eye should be left in place, supported with a doughnut dressing, and secured with a gauze dressing. Since both eyes move together, the uninjured eye should also be covered to prevent sympathetic movement. (ECTSI 5, pp. 354–357)

13: **B.** A crushing injury of the neck may result in a fractured larynx. (ECTSI 5, p. 367)

14: **D.** Avulsed tissue of the ear, scalp, or nose should be recovered, placed in a moist, sterile dressing in a plastic bag, kept cool, and transported to the hospital with the patient. (ECTSI 5, p. 365)

15: **C.** Both eyes should be covered when treating a patient with an injury to one eye to prevent sympathetic movement. (ECTSI 5, p. 354)

16: **D.** Cerebrospinal fluid acts as a shock absorber for the brain and spinal cord. (ECTSI 5, p. 320)

17: **C.** The only emergency treatment for chemical burns to the eye is flushing the eye with water or sterile saline solution. (ECTSI 5, p. 357)

18: **D.** Maintain the airway of an unconscious patient with a head injury by stabilizing the head and cervical spine in a neutral, in-line position. (ECTSI 5, p. 328)

19: **B.** Chemical burns to the eyes should be irrigated with clean water or sterile saline solution for at least 20 minutes. In this case, it may be appropriate to provide continuous irrigation en route to the hospital. (ECTSI 5, p. 357)

20: **B.** If cerebrospinal fluid is leaking from the ear, nose, or scalp, cover them loosely to prevent contamination. (ECTSI 5, p. 332)

21: **A.** An unconscious patient with a head injury may have brain damage if the pupils of the eyes are unequal. (ECTSI 5, p. 332)

22: **B.** Removal of a foreign object that penetrates the cheek into the mouth may be necessary if it could cause further injury or possibly obstruct the airway. To stop the bleeding in this type of injury, hold gauze against both the inside and outside of the cheek. (ECTSI 5, p. 364)

23: **D.** You should look for another serious injury. Low blood pressure or shock rarely result from the head injury itself. (ECTSI 5, p. 329)

24: **B.** The first step in caring for a patient with a throat injury is to ensure that the patient's airway is clear. (ECTSI 5, p. 367)

Injuries of the Head, Eyes, Mouth, and Face

25: **D.** A patient who is unconscious immediately after an accident, then regains consciousness, may have a closed head injury, such as a concussion. (ECTSI 5, p. 324)

26: **C.** The meninges consist of the dura mater, arachnoid, and the pia mater. These three layers surround and protect the brain and the spinal cord. (ECTSI 5, p. 320)

27: **A.** The spinal cord is considered a continuation of the brainstem. (ECTSI 5, p. 315)

28: **A.** The dura mater is a protective covering for the brain. (ECTSI 5, p. 320)

29: **C.** With head injuries, level of consciousness often fluctuates. The patient's level of consciousness should be monitored during transport to the hospital. (ECTSI 5, pp. 327, 330)

30: **B.** The face and scalp are said to be vascular because they are well supplied with arteries and veins. (ECTSI 5, p. 364)

31: **C.** The first step in treating a bleeding head wound should consist of local manual pressure with a dry, sterile dressing. (ECTSI 5, p. 330)

32: **B.** A foreign object impaled in the skull should be left in place, but should be stabilized with a bulky dressing. (ECTSI 5, pp. 238–239)

33: **A.** An unconscious patient with facial injuries should be properly immobilized and then transported in a side-lying position to aid in airway management. (ECTSI 5, p. 365)

34: **A.** As long as the globe is not damaged in a laceration injury of the eyelid, there may be no permanent vision loss. (ECTSI 5, p. 359)

35: **D.** Because there is little room for expansion of the brain within the skull, swelling of the brain (cerebral edema) is a serious condition. (ECTSI 5, pp. 325–326)

36: **D.** Airway obstruction is a constant risk for patients with facial fractures. (ECTSI 5, pp. 366–367)

37: **A.** Discoloration of the soft tissues around the eye as a result of a head injury is called ecchymosis, or raccoon eyes. Battle's sign is ecchymosis behind the ear. (ECTSI 5, p. 324)

Chapter 14

38: **D.** The AVPU scale (Alert, Verbal, Pain, Unresponsive) provides a baseline evaluation of a patient's level of consciousness. Reevaluations should be done every 10 minutes until the patient reaches the hospital. (ECTSI 5, p. 327)

39: **D.** Supplemental oxygen should always be given routinely to a patient who has a head injury. Supplemental oxygen is needed to restore the inadequate oxygenation of the blood and prevent swelling of the brain (cerebral edema). (ECTSI 5, p. 328)

Chapter 15

Injuries and Problems of the Chest, Abdomen, and Genitalia

Chapter Goals

The exercises in this chapter are designed to help the student to:

- identify the signs and symptoms of chest injury.

- describe the differences between tension pneumothorax, sucking chest wound, flail chest, and traumatic asphyxia.

- describe the serious chest problems that can occur spontaneously without trauma.

- identify the signs and symptoms of an acute abdomen.

- list the organs in the abdomen and identify their correct location.

- describe common injuries of the male and female genitalia.

- explain how to control bleeding of the genitalia.

Chapter 15

Multiple-Choice Questions

Select the correct answer for each of the following questions. Each question has only *one* correct or best answer.

1. Immediate care for a patient with an acute abdomen includes giving the patient:

    A. an antacid for pain relief.

    B. an analgesic for pain relief.

    C. plenty of water to drink.

    D. nothing to eat or drink.

2. A patient who has pain and tenderness in the right upper quadrant of the abdomen, but no history of injury, may have:

    A. appendicitis.

    B. a ruptured spleen.

    C. gallbladder disease.

    D. an aortic aneursym.

3. A patient who has pain and tenderness in the left upper quadrant of the abdomen as a result of injury may have:

    A. appendicitis.

    B. a ruptured spleen.

    C. pancreatitis.

    D. gallbladder disease.

4. In which quadrant is most of the stomach located?

    A. Right upper

    B. Right lower

    C. Left upper

    D. Left lower

Injuries and Problems of the Chest, Abdomen, and Genitalia

5. The liver is located in the:

   A. right upper quadrant, beneath the diaphragm.

   B. right upper quadrant, beneath the stomach.

   C. left upper quadrant, beneath the diaphragm.

   D. left upper quadrant, beneath the stomach.

6. A patient with a sucking chest wound has a sudden drop in blood pressure and pulse, and deteriorating respirations after an occlusive dressing is applied. You should first:

   A. give high-flow oxygen.

   B. apply a second dressing on top of the first.

   C. place the patient in a side-lying position to prevent choking.

   D. release one edge of the dressing to allow air to escape.

7. A 23-year-old man has a sudden, sharp chest pain, along with increasing difficulty breathing. His lungs are clear, although lung sounds on the left side are somewhat diminished. There is no sign of an open wound on the chest. Your care of this patient should begin by:

   A. performing CPR.

   B. clearing and maintaining the airway.

   C. wrapping the chest with occlusive dressings.

   D. encouraging the patient to cough and then take deep breaths.

8. Which of the following is a common sign of an acute abdomen?

   A. Diarrhea

   B. High blood pressure

   C. Low body temperature

   D. Rapid, shallow breathing

Chapter 15

9. The most effective way to help a conscious patient with a flail chest to breathe more easily is to:

   A. insert an oropharyngeal airway.

   B. give supplemental oxygen.

   C. give mouth-to-mouth ventilations.

   D. seal the wound with an occlusive dressing.

10. A 30-year-old man who was pinned under an automobile for several minutes has now been removed by the rescue team. The patient is cyanotic, and has rapid, shallow breathing. You notice that each time the patient breathes in, the chest wall moves inward rather than outward. These signs suggest that the patient may have a:

    A. flail chest.

    B. hemothorax.

    C. pneumothorax.

    D. ruptured main stem bronchus.

11. The accumulation of blood, fluid, or air in the chest cavity can result in:

    A. increased lung volume.

    B. decreased lung volume.

    C. hypertension.

    D. a flail chest.

12. A man has difficulty breathing after an automobile accident. The area around his lips and tongue is blue, and the area around his head and shoulders is dark blue. His eyes are bloodshot and appear to be bulging. These signs and symptoms suggest:

    A. subcutaneous emphysema.

    B. traumatic asphyxia.

    C. tension pneumothorax.

    D. spontaneous pneumothorax.

Injuries and Problems of the Chest, Abdomen, and Genitalia

13. The term *hemothorax* means that:

    A. air is continuously leaking from the lung into the pleural space.

    B. blood is collecting in the chest cavity within the pleural space.

    C. blood is leaking into the pericardial sac.

    D. blood is pooling in the airway.

14. A patient has a large laceration on the abdomen, and the intestines appear to protrude through the wound. You should first cover the intestines with:

    A. absorbent cotton.

    B. a dry, sterile dressing.

    C. moistened, sterile dressings.

    D. saline-soaked dressings, then gently try to place them back into the abdomen.

15. The urinary bladder is located in the:

    A. pelvic cavity behind the pubic bone.

    B. abdominal cavity below the diaphragm.

    C. abdominal cavity below the stomach.

    D. thoracic cavity below the left lung.

16. Which of the following structures is located within the thoracic cavity?

    A. Spleen

    B. Scapula

    C. Esophagus

    D. Gallbladder

Chapter 15

17. Which of the following signs and symptoms most commonly appear in a patient who has acute appendicitis?

    A. Pain and tenderness in the right lower quadrant

    B. Pain and tenderness in the left lower quadrant

    C. Pain in the upper quadrants, tenderness in the abdomen

    D. Cramps in the right upper quadrant

18. An impaled object in the abdomen should be:

    A. removed carefully if the patient is thrashing about.

    B. removed carefully and direct manual pressure applied.

    C. left in place and stabilized with aluminum foil.

    D. left in place and stabilized with soft roller gauze.

19. The first step in caring for a patient who has a penetrating chest wound is to:

    A. provide rapid transport.

    B. secure the airway.

    C. control any external bleeding.

    D. elevate the feet to prevent shock.

20. A patient with a blunt abdominal injury should be transported in what position?

    A. Supine with the head turned to one side

    B. Supine with the head flexed

    C. Side-lying with the head flexed

    D. Prone with the head turned to one side

21. The crackling sensation produced by air bubbles escaping from the lungs into surrounding tissues after a chest wound is called:

    A. a flail chest.

    B. pneumothorax.

    C. traumatic asphyxia.

    D. subcutaneous emphysema.

Injuries and Problems of the Chest, Abdomen, and Genitalia

22. Vomit that contains bright red blood or has a texture like coffee grounds suggests possible:

    A. gastrointestinal bleeding.

    B. rupture of the spleen.

    C. puncture of the lung.

    D. rupture of the aorta.

23. Assessment of a patient with a chest injury is most likely to reveal:

    A. a slow, weak pulse.

    B. high blood pressure.

    C. difficulty breathing and pain at the site of the injury.

    D. pale yellow discoloration of the lips and fingernails.

24. Initial emergency care of a patient with an acute abdomen should include:

    A. administering a mild sedative.

    B. clearing and maintaining the airway.

    C. giving the patient small sips of water.

    D. administering epinephrine to prevent anaphylactic shock.

25. What is your primary responsibility for a patient who has signs and symptoms of an acute abdomen?

    A. Determining the exact cause of the pain

    B. Ensuring the patient drinks plenty of water

    C. Giving the patient an analgesic for pain relief

    D. Providing prompt transport to the hospital

Chapter 15

26. A man is involved in an automobile accident in which the steering column collapses. You assess the patient's ABCs and provide manual stabilization of the spine. You should next assess for:

    A. a flail chest.

    B. a fractured femur.

    C. ruptured kidneys.

    D. fractured vertebrae.

27. Which of the following abdominal organs is hollow?

    A. Liver

    B. Spleen

    C. Pancreas

    D. Gallbladder

28. Which of the following abdominal organs is solid?

    A. Kidney

    B. Duodenum

    C. Appendix

    D. Urinary bladder

29. A patient with a flail chest has difficulty breathing because the:

    A. air pressure in the lungs is increased.

    B. air pressure in the lungs is constant.

    C. lung beneath the flail segment is punctured.

    D. lung beneath the flail segment cannot expand properly.

Injuries and Problems of the Chest, Abdomen, and Genitalia

30. A construction worker has a severe compression injury to the chest after a ceiling falls on him. The patient appears to have multiple rib fractures and a possible flail chest segment. During assessment you note that the patient's neck veins are distended, and the upper part of his body is turning blue. Your first step in caring for this patient is to:

    A. elevate the feet.

    B. place him in a side-lying position.

    C. apply an occlusive dressing to the chest wound.

    D. give him supplemental oxygen and assist ventilations, if necessary.

31. The "sucking" sound characteristic of certain open chest wounds occurs because as the patient breathes:

    A. air passes in and out of the heart.

    B. air passes in and out of the wound.

    C. muscles around the wound tear.

    D. blood pools in and around the lungs.

32. The most appropriate way to prevent air from entering an open chest wound is to:

    A. seal the wound with an occlusive dressing.

    B. pack the wound with thick dressings.

    C. tape a small pillow over the wound.

    D. tape the wound closed with absorbent cotton.

33. Paradoxical movement of the chest means that as the patient breathes, the loose chest section:

    A. remains still as the rest of the chest wall moves in and out.

    B. moves opposite to the movement of the rest of the chest wall.

    C. changes size as the rest of the chest wall moves in and out.

    D. moves in and out with the rest of the chest wall.

Chapter 15

34. The presence of blood in the urine is known as:

    A. hematochezia.

    B. hematemesis.

    C. hematoma.

    D. hematuria.

35. Initial treatment to control bleeding from the female genitalia should include:

    A. packing and placing dressings in the vagina.

    B. applying dry, sterile compresses, and local pressure.

    C. applying moist, sterile compresses, and local pressure.

    D. removing any impaled objects and applying local pressure.

36. Initial treatment to control bleeding from the male genitalia should include:

    A. applying local pressure with a sterile dressing.

    B. providing immediate transport to the hospital.

    C. placing the patient in a supine position with the legs elevated.

    D. irrigating the injury with sterile saline solution.

37. Injuries to either the male or female genitalia are most likely to result in:

    A. little or no pain.

    B. great anxiety to the patient.

    C. a threat to the patient's life.

    D. little or no bleeding.

38. Emergency treatment of a direct blow to the scrotum should include:

    A. placing the patient in a supine position and providing immediate transport.

    B. placing the patient in a prone position and providing immediate transport.

    C. applying cold dressings during transport.

    D. applying moist, sterile dressings during transport.

Injuries and Problems of the Chest, Abdomen, and Genitalia

39. An object impaled in the male or female external genitalia should be:

    A. removed in an attempt to stop bleeding with local pressure.

    B. removed to make the patient more comfortable.

    C. left in place but adjusted for the patient's comfort before stabilizing with bandages.

    D. left in place and stabilized with bandages.

40. A man has an avulsion injury to the penis, and the avulsed tissue has not been located. Before transporting the patient to the hospital, you should:

    A. wrap the denuded part with a moist, sterile dressing and quickly attempt to find and preserve the avulsed tissue.

    B. wrap the denuded part with a dry, sterile dressing and quickly attempt to find and preserve the avulsed tissue.

    C. spend as much time as necessary to find the avulsed tissue, wash it with sterile saline solution, replace it onto its bed, and wrap the part with moist, sterile dressings.

    D. spend as much time as necessary to find the avulsed tissue, place it into a plastic bag filled with ice, and loosely bandage the part.

Answers

1: **D.** Under no circumstances should you give a patient with acute abdominal signs anything to eat or drink. (ECTSI 5, p. 496)

2: **C.** Pain and tenderness without injury in the right upper quadrant of the abdomen often indicates gallbladder disease. (ECTSI 5, p. 57)

3: **B.** Pain and tenderness in the left upper quadrant of the abdomen following injury often indicates a ruptured spleen. (ECTSI 5, p. 58)

4: **C.** Most of the stomach is located in the left upper quadrant of the abdomen. (ECTSI 5, p. 57)

5: **A.** The liver lies primarily in the right upper quadrant, beneath the diaphragm. (ECTSI 5, p. 57)

Chapter 15

6: **D.** Deteriorating breathing, weakening pulse, and falling blood pressure are signs of a tension pneumothorax. Other signs include bulging of the tissues of the chest wall between the ribs and above the clavicle, distention of the neck veins, and cyanosis. Your first step in caring for a patient with these signs and symptoms is to release one edge of the dressing to allow the air under tension to escape. (ECTSI 5, p. 381)

7: **B.** Signs of a spontaneous pneumothorax include sudden sharp chest pain and shortness of breath. Your first steps in caring for this patient should be clearing and maintaining the airway, followed by giving oxygen, and providing transport. (ECTSI 5, p. 380)

8: **D.** Rapid, shallow breathing is a common sign of an acute abdomen. (ECTSI 5, p. 492)

9: **B.** To help a patient with a flail chest breathe easier, give supplemental oxygen. (ECTSI 5, p. 378)

10: **A.** Paradoxical motion of the chest, and in some patients, cyanosis and hypoxia indicate a flail chest. (ECTSI 5, p. 377)

11: **B.** The accumulation of blood, fluid, or air in the chest cavity can cause lung volume to decrease. (ECTSI 5, pp. 379–382)

12: **B.** Common signs of traumatic asphyxia include cyanosis and swelling of the upper body, distended neck veins, and bloodshot, bulging eyes. (ECTSI 5, p. 379)

13: **B.** Hemothorax is the presence of blood collecting in the chest cavity within the pleural space. (ECTSI 5, pp. 381–382)

14: **C.** Cover an abdominal evisceration with a sterile gauze dressing moistened with sterile saline solution, and then secure it with sterile aluminum foil. (ECTSI 5, p. 406)

15: **A.** The urinary bladder is located in the pelvic cavity behind the pubic bone. (ECTSI 5, p. 397)

16: **C.** The esophagus is located in the thoracic cavity. (ECTSI 5, p. 55)

17: **A.** The appendix is located in the right lower quadrant. Pain and tenderness in this region may be caused by appendicitis. (ECTSI 5, p. 58)

Injuries and Problems of the Chest, Abdomen, and Genitalia

18: **D.** With an impalement injury to the abdomen, you should leave the object in place and apply a stabilizing bandage of soft roller gauze to control bleeding and prevent movement of the object. (ECTSI 5, p. 406)

19: **B.** The first step in caring for a patient who has a penetrating chest injury is to secure and maintain the patient's airway. Supplemental oxygen should then be given and the patient's feet elevated to prevent hypovolemic shock. (ECTSI 5, p. 379)

20: **A.** A patient with a blunt abdominal injury should be transported in a supine position with the head turned to one side. (ECTSI 5, p. 404)

21: **D.** With subcutaneous emphysema, small air bubbles lie in the subcutaneous tissues of the chest wall after an injury, resulting in a definite crackling sensation under the skin on palpation. (ECTSI 5, p. 383)

22: **A.** Vomiting of bright red blood or blood with a coffee grounds texture suggests possible gastrointestinal bleeding. (ECTSI 5, pp. 501–502)

23: **C.** Assessment of a patient with a chest injury is most likely to reveal difficulty breathing and pain at the site of the injury. (ECTSI 5, pp. 373–374)

24: **B.** Initial emergency care of a patient with an acute abdomen should include clearing and maintaining the patient's airway. (ECTSI 5, p. 496)

25: **D.** Your primary responsibility to a patient who has acute abdominal pain is to provide prompt transport to the hospital. Never give any food, fluids, or pain medication to a patient with acute abdominal pain. The patient may require surgery, and the presence of food in the stomach may make the surgery more dangerous. Pain medication may mask important signs and symptoms. (ECTSI 5, p. 496)

26: **A.** In this situation, you should first assess the patient's ABCs and then provide manual stabilization of the spine. Only then should you proceed to assess for a flail chest. (ECTSI 5, pp. 376–378)

27: **D.** The gallbladder is a hollow organ. (ECTSI 5, p. 390)

28: **A.** The kidney is a solid organ. (ECTSI 5, p. 390)

29: **D.** A patient with a flail chest has difficulty breathing because the lung immediately beneath the flail segment cannot expand properly during inhalation. (ECTSI 5, pp. 376–378)

Chapter 15

30: **D.** A compression injury to the chest resulting in multiple rib fractures and a flail chest may lead to traumatic asphyxia. Therefore, your first step in caring for the patient is to provide vigorous respiratory support and prompt transport to the hospital. (ECTSI 5, p. 379)

31: **B.** The characteristic "sucking" sound occurs when air passes in and out of the wound. (ECTSI 5, pp. 382–383)

32: **A.** Appropriate treatment of an open chest wound should include sealing the wound with an occlusive dressing. (ECTSI 5, pp. 382–383)

33: **B.** When paradoxical movement of the chest occurs in a flail chest injury, the loose chest section moves in the direction opposite to the movement of the rest of the chest wall. (ECTSI 5, pp. 376–378)

34: **D.** The presence of blood in the urine is known as hematuria. (ECTSI 5, p. 407)

35: **C.** The most appropriate way to control bleeding of a wound to the female genitalia is to apply moist, sterile compresses, local pressure, and a diaper-type bandage to hold the dressings in place. (ECTSI 5, p. 410)

36: **A.** The most appropriate way to control bleeding of a wound to the male genitalia is to apply local pressure with a sterile dressing. (ECTSI 5, pp. 408–409)

37: **B.** Injuries to both male and female genitalia may bleed profusely, and be very painful, but they are not usually immediately life threatening. These injuries, however, result in great anxiety to the patient. (ECTSI 5, pp. 408–410)

38: **C.** Appropriate treatment for a patient who sustained a direct blow to the scrotum should include application of cold dressings during transport to the hospital. (ECTSI 5, p. 409)

39: **D.** An object impaled in the male or female external genitalia should be left in place and stabilized with bandages. (ECTSI 5, p. 410)

40: **A.** Before transporting a patient with an avulsion injury to the penis, you should wrap the denuded part with a moist, sterile dressing and quickly attempt to find and preserve the avulsed tissue. (ECTSI 5, pp. 408–409)

Chapter 16

General Medical Emergencies

Chapter Goals

The exercises in this chapter are designed to help the student to:

- describe the signs and symptoms of various heart conditions, such as angina pectoris, acute myocardial infarction, congestive heart failure.

- explain the steps in proper emergency care of various heart conditions, such as angina pectoris, acute myocardial infarction, congestive heart failure.

- describe the signs and symptoms of a cerebrovascular accident.

- compare the signs and symptoms of insulin shock with diabetic coma.

- explain the steps in proper emergency care of diabetic emergencies.

- describe the signs and symptoms of breathing difficulties, including asthma, hyperventilation, and chronic obstructive pulmonary disease (COPD).

- identify common communicable diseases and infectious processes.

- explain how to minimize the risk of transmission of communicable diseases.

- describe proper emergency treatment of epilepsy and convulsions.

- explain how to assess for the various causes of unconsciousness.

Chapter 16

Multiple-Choice Questions

Select the correct answer for each of the following questions. Each question has only *one* correct or best answer.

1. You arrive at the home of a woman who is found lying on the floor convulsing. Your first step in caring for this woman is to:

    A. insert a bite stick, with force if needed.

    B. give her oxygen by face mask.

    C. insert an oropharyngeal airway.

    D. clear the area surrounding the woman to protect her from injury.

2. A patient who has a history of epilepsy just experienced a seizure episode, but appears to have no injuries. The patient should be advised to:

    A. take aspirin.

    B. take a short walk.

    C. drink coffee or cola.

    D. try to sleep or rest.

3. What is the principal difference between a generalized seizure and a partial seizure?

    A. In a generalized seizure, most of the brain is affected by abnormal electrical activity.

    B. In a generalized seizure, seizure activity is limited to one side of the body.

    C. Unconsciousness usually occurs with a partial seizure.

    D. A partial seizure has three distinct phases: aura, convulsion, and postictal state.

General Medical Emergencies

4. An unconscious woman has unequal pupils and her left side appears to be paralyzed. There is no history of trauma or head injury. The patient should be transported to the hospital on her:

   A. back with her feet slightly elevated.

   B. back with her head slightly elevated.

   C. side with her head slightly lower than her feet.

   D. side with her head slightly higher than her feet.

5. A young man who has just been fighting with his boss has rapid, deep respirations, dizziness, numbness around the mouth, and tingling fingers. Proper care for this patient should consist of:

   A. instructing him to breathe into a paper bag.

   B. giving supplemental oxygen.

   C. providing reassurance and transport to the hospital.

   D. clearing the surrounding area in preparation for a seizure.

6. Unconsciousness may quickly occur in which of the following conditions associated with diabetes?

   A. Insulin shock

   B. Diabetic coma

   C. Polyuria

   D. Hyperglycemia

7. Fluid sounds in the lungs without trauma may indicate:

   A. shock.

   B. stroke.

   C. diabetic emergency.

   D. cardiac emergency.

American Academy of Orthopaedic Surgeons

Chapter 16

8. An elderly woman is having difficulty breathing even though her head is elevated with two pillows. Her ankles are swollen, and when you gently press on her ankle, your finger leaves a depression on the skin. As you prepare the patient for transport, you should:

    A. give her oxygen and elevate her feet and legs.

    B. give her oxygen and transport her in a sitting position.

    C. apply air splints to both legs to force blood back to the heart.

    D. place her in a prone position with her head slightly elevated.

9. In what two principal ways does the pain from acute myocardial infarction (AMI) differ from the pain of angina?

    A. With AMI, the pain lasts longer and is not related to emotional stress or exercise.

    B. With AMI, the pain lasts longer, but is relieved by medication.

    C. With AMI, the pain lasts only a short time and is often caused by emotional stress or exercise.

    D. With AMI, the pain can be sudden, but is readily relieved with rest.

10. A 39-year-old man has pain to the left of his sternum immediately after playing touch football with his children. Thirty minutes later, his family calls because he is shaken and still in pain. You should transport the patient to the hospital due to possible:

    A. angina pectoris.

    B. myocardial infarction.

    C. congestive heart failure.

    D. spontaneous pneumothorax.

11. A 54-year-old woman suddenly collapses outside a theater. Her pupils are dilated, and she has no detectable pulse or respirations. A Medic-Alert bracelet on her arm states that she is a diabetic. You should prepare to treat the patient for:

    A. stroke.

    B. insulin shock.

    C. diabetic coma.

    D. cardiac arrest.

General Medical Emergencies

12. Which of the following conditions is characterized by inadequate pumping action of the heart, resulting in fluid buildup in the body?

    A. Stroke

    B. Angina pectoris

    C. Bradycardia

    D. Congestive heart failure

13. You can help a conscious patient to take a prescribed nitroglycerin pill by making sure that the patient:

    A. places the pill under his tongue.

    B. swallows the pill with a full glass of water.

    C. swallows the pill with a full glass of milk.

    D. chews the pill completely before swallowing.

14. A man has severe chest pain shortly after he stopped working in the yard. Upon your arrival 10 minutes later, the pain seems less severe, but the patient states that his chest felt as if it were being squeezed in a vise. Your first step in caring for this patient would be to:

    A. give supplemental oxygen.

    B. reassure the patient that you are there to help him.

    C. obtain and record the patient's vital signs.

    D. provide immediate transport.

15. You are preparing to transport a woman believed to have had an acute myocardial infarction. She denies that she has "had a heart attack," but offers to get into the ambulance to go to the hospital. The most appropriate course of action would be to:

    A. allow her to walk from her bed to the stretcher.

    B. allow her to walk from the house into the ambulance.

    C. assist her in walking from the house into the ambulance.

    D. transfer her to the stretcher, elevate the head of the stretcher, and give her oxygen en route to the hospital.

Chapter 16

16. A 65-year-old man who has a history of heart disease suddenly becomes tired and begins to sweat profusely. These findings suggest:

    A. angina pectoris.

    B. myocardial infarction.

    C. congestive heart failure.

    D. a cerebrovascular accident.

17. A weakened, dilated portion of an artery is called:

    A. a thrombus.

    B. an aneurysm.

    C. an embolus.

    D. an occlusion.

18. The pain that occurs with a heart attack is due to:

    A. anxiety.

    B. arrhythmia.

    C. decreased oxygen supply to the heart.

    D. decreased nutrient supply to the heart.

19. A patient believed to be having an acute myocardial infarction has substernal pain and is cyanotic. He states that he "cannot be having a heart attack. I have emphysema." You have been giving him supplemental oxygen at 4 L/min, but he is still cyanotic. The next step in caring for this patient should include:

    A. rebreathing into a paper bag.

    B. reducing the oxygen flow.

    C. inserting an airway and ventilating with positive pressure.

    D. increasing the oxygen flow, but preparing to assist with ventilation.

General Medical Emergencies

20. What is the best way to give supplemental oxygen to a patient with chronic obstructive pulmonary disease (COPD)?

    A. Venturi mask

    B. Nasal cannula

    C. Simple face mask

    D. Nonrebreathing mask

21. A 51-year-old woman lying on a sofa is unable to sit up without help. She cannot describe how she feels because her speech is slurred and incoherent. Her hand grasps are unequal, and you note that she is drooling. After you check her airway, you should next:

    A. check the pulse at the wrist and the neck.

    B. give the patient water to clear her throat.

    C. place the patient in a side-lying position for transport.

    D. help the patient to her feet and assist her with walking around.

22. Which of the following findings is most commonly associated with a cerebrovascular accident?

    A. Unequal pupils

    B. Stiffness in the neck

    C. Paralysis of the lower extremities

    D. Paralysis of one side of the body

23. Nitroglycerin is most often prescribed as treatment of:

    A. angina pectoris.

    B. acute myocardial infarction.

    C. congestive heart failure.

    D. cerebrovascular accident.

Chapter 16

24. Supplemental oxygen must be given carefully to a patient who has chronic obstructive pulmonary disease (COPD) because a rapid rise in arterial oxygen may:

    A. result in severe chest pain.

    B. cause oxygen intoxication.

    C. shut down the patient's oxygen drive and eventually cause respiratory arrest.

    D. make the accessory muscles of the neck and shoulder work harder, making breathing more difficult for the patient.

25. Blockage in the coronary artery causes which of the following conditions?

    A. Stroke

    B. Angina pectoris

    C. Myocardial infarction

    D. Congestive heart failure

26. Nitroglycerin acts to relieve cardiac pain by:

    A. deadening the pain sensation.

    B. decreasing blood flow to the heart.

    C. dilating the coronary arteries.

    D. increasing blood pressure.

27. A 35-year-old woman who appears to be going into insulin shock is still conscious, but is becoming pale and sweaty. Your immediate treatment should include giving the patient:

    A. sips of fruit juice.

    B. sips of water.

    C. a candy bar.

    D. intravenous fluids and insulin.

General Medical Emergencies

28. Insulin causes blood sugar (glucose) to be:

    A. produced.

    B. able to enter the cells.

    C. able to enter the liver.

    D. removed from the cells.

29. What is the principal physiologic difference between type I and type II diabetes?

    A. With type I diabetes, a person produces too much insulin.

    B. With type I diabetes, a person does not produce adequate insulin.

    C. With type II diabetes, a person needs an insulin injection every day.

    D. With type II diabetes, a person has had the disease since childhood.

30. What are the two most important questions to ask a conscious patient who is experiencing a diabetic emergency?

    A. "How do you feel?" and "Can you breathe easy?"

    B. "How old are you?" and "What kind of diabetes do you have?"

    C. "Have you taken insulin today?" and "Have you eaten today?"

    D. "Can you talk?" and "What kind of diabetes do you have?"

31. A young man is drifting in and out of consciousness due to either insulin shock or diabetic coma. Because you are not sure of the cause of the patient's condition, you should:

    A. give the patient sugar.

    B. give the patient a glass of juice.

    C. ask the patient about his condition when he appears awake.

    D. provide prompt transport to the hospital.

Chapter 16

32. An excess of insulin, due to too much insulin production, failure to eat, or over-exercise, causes which of the following conditions?

    A. Pancreatitis

    B. Insulin shock

    C. Diabetic coma

    D. Gluconeogenesis

33. Sweet, fruity breath is a common sign of which of the following conditions associated with diabetes?

    A. Insulin shock

    B. Diabetic ketoacidosis

    C. Hyperglycemia

    D. Polydipsia

34. Treatment of asthma should include providing the patient with:

    A. a paper bag for rebreathing.

    B. supplemental oxygen for easier breathing.

    C. a nasopharyngeal airway for easier breathing.

    D. an oropharyngeal airway for easier breathing.

35. A spontaneous pneumothorax is best described as:

    A. a very severe compression of the chest.

    B. the presence of blood in the chest cavity.

    C. a rupture of the lung that allows air into the pleural space.

    D. air leaking from the lungs that eventually collects under the skin.

General Medical Emergencies

36. Which of the following emergency care measures is **NOT** appropriate for a patient who has emphysema?

    A. Transporting the patient in a sitting position

    B. Explaining what you are going to do to help the patient

    C. Helping the patient to take his or her prescribed medication

    D. Giving the patient supplemental oxygen at a high flow rate

37. A patient experiencing asthma asks you to help her with her emergency epinephrine kit. An appropriate response to her request would be:

    A. "I am not able to help give medications. You need to wait until you get to the hospital."

    B. "I have an emergency epinephrine kit in the ambulance. We will not need to use yours."

    C. "You don't need to take any medication. Try breathing into this paper bag."

    D. "Tell me where your medication is and I will help you to take it."

38. Which of the following conditions is characterized by spasm and constriction of the bronchial tubes, resulting in congestion and difficulty in breathing?

    A. Asthma

    B. Asphyxia

    C. Pneumonia

    D. Emphysema

39. Of the following, which condition is **NOT** considered a communicable disease?

    A. Mumps

    B. Measles

    C. Emphysema

    D. Chickenpox

Chapter 16

40. Proper disposal of sharps includes which of the following steps?

    A. Recapping and then placing in a sharps container

    B. Cutting in two and then placing in a sharps container

    C. Rinsing with alcohol, recapping, then placing in a sharps container

    D. Placing in a sharps container immediately after use without rinsing, recapping, or cutting

41. Transmission of tuberculosis most commonly occurs through contact with an infected person's:

    A. blood.

    B. clothing.

    C. semen.

    D. sputum.

42. A PPD skin test is performed on EMTs prior to employment to check for exposure to:

    A. AIDS.

    B. hepatitis B.

    C. meningitis.

    D. tuberculosis.

43. Which of the following measures is **NOT** considered proper body substance isolation for the EMT when caring for a patient believed to have a communicable disease?

    A. Changing gloves between patients at a mass-casualty incident

    B. Rinsing and recapping needles before disposal in an appropriate sharps container

    C. Wearing a gown when your uniform may become extensively soiled with blood or other body fluids

    D. Wearing both protective eyewear and a face mask when blood or other body fluids may splatter

General Medical Emergencies

44. Which of the following situations presents the greatest opportunity for acquiring a communicable disease?

    A. You have eaten "spoiled" lobster.

    B. You are bitten by a mosquito outside the hospital.

    C. You hear the patient coughing in the back of the ambulance.

    D. You clean the back of the ambulance after a "bloody run" with a bleach and water mixture using your bare hands.

45. You should check for bracelets or necklaces on unconscious patients in order to learn:

    A. the patient's name and address.

    B. the name of the patient's physician.

    C. information about the patient's insurance status.

    D. information about possible medical problems.

46. You are called to a bar where you find a semiconscious man lying on the floor. He appears to be intoxicated. The most appropriate course of action would be to:

    A. call the police to handle the matter.

    B. tell bystanders to take the patient home.

    C. perform a thorough assessment and transport.

    D. take the patient home and tell him to "sleep it off."

47. What is the first step in caring for an unconscious patient, after ensuring that the patient is breathing and not in any danger?

    A. Placing the patient on his or her back

    B. Determining level of responsiveness

    C. Elevating the patient's feet

    D. Tilting the head back

Chapter 16

Answers

1: **D.** You should first clear the area surrounding the woman to protect her from additional injury. You should not try to insert a bite stick, as you may break her teeth, or the stick may be bitten in two and cause airway obstruction. (ECTSI 5, p. 552)

2: **D.** A patient with a history of epilepsy will also have a history of seizures. Very often the seizure episode will make the patient tired. If the patient is not injured, you should advise the patient to try to sleep or rest, not to walk around or take any kind of medication. (ECTSI 5, p. 552)

3: **A.** In a generalized seizure, most of the brain is involved in the abnormal electrical discharge. Usually all extremities are involved in the muscular activity, and the patient becomes unconscious. (ECTSI 5, p. 550)

4: **D.** An unconscious patient who has no history of trauma or head injury and has an open airway should be transported in a side-lying position, with the head slightly higher (6 inches) than the feet. (ECTSI 5, pp. 463–464)

5. **C.** Dizziness, numbness around the mouth, and a tingling sensation in the extremities, along with the difficulty in breathing, suggests hyperventilation. Traditionally, breathing into a paper bag has been the treatment of choice. However, this method may not be effective, because the blood carbon dioxide level does not rise significantly. Therefore, provide reassurance and transport the patient to the emergency department. (ECTSI 5, p. 478)

6: **A.** Unconsciousness may develop quickly with insulin shock. (ECTSI 5, pp. 486, 546)

7: **D.** Of the conditions listed, only a cardiac emergency would cause fluid sounds in the lungs. (ECTSI 5, p. 455)

8: **B.** This patient has signs of chronic congestive heart failure and should be given oxygen and transported in a sitting position. (ECTSI 5, p. 456)

9: **A.** The two principal ways in which the pain of angina pectoris and acute myocardial infarction (AMI) differ are duration and cause. With AMI, the pain lasts longer and is not related to emotional stress or exercise. (ECTSI 5, p. 452)

10: **B.** A first episode at age 39 with continued pain suggests myocardial infarction. (ECTSI 5, p. 452)

General Medical Emergencies

11: **D.** The absence of pulse and respirations in this patient indicates cardiac arrest. (ECTSI 5, p. 111)

12: **D.** Inadequate pumping of the heart that results in fluid buildup is indicative of congestive heart failure. (ECTSI 5, p. 455)

13: **A.** You can help a conscious patient to take a prescribed nitroglycerin pill by making sure that the patient places the pill under his tongue. (ECTSI 5, p. 450)

14: **B.** Your first step in caring for this patient is to reassure him that you are there to help him. Oftentimes, patients who experience angina or acute myocardial infarction will be very anxious, or will deny that they have a heart condition. Therefore, your first step with all such patients is to reassure them. (ECTSI 5, p. 454)

15: **D.** A patient believed to have had a heart attack should not be allowed to lift his or her own weight. Therefore, your most appropriate action in this situation would be to transfer the patient to a stretcher, elevate the head of the stretcher, and give her oxygen en route to the hospital. (ECTSI 5, p. 453)

16: **B.** These signs and symptoms and the patient's history suggest possible myocardial infarction. (ECTSI 5, p. 452)

17: **B.** A weakened, dilated portion of an artery is called an aneurysm. (ECTSI 5, p. 461)

18: **C.** The pain of a heart attack is due to a decreased supply of blood and oxygen to the heart muscle. (ECTSI 5, p. 449)

19: **D.** In this situation, you should increase the oxygen flow, but be prepared to assist with ventilation should respiratory arrest occur. (ECTSI 5, p. 475)

20: **A.** The preferred way to give supplemental oxygen to a patient with chronic obstructive pulmonary disease (COPD) is via a Venturi mask. (ECTSI 5, p. 475)

21: **A.** The patient's signs and symptoms suggest a cerebrovascular accident. Your first priority is to make sure the airway is clear. The next step in caring for the patient is to check the pulse at the wrist and at the neck. Monitoring the carotid pulse could be helpful to the physician. (ECTSI 5, pp. 462–463)

Chapter 16

22: **D.** Paralysis of one side of the body commonly occurs as a result of a cerebrovascular accident. (ECTSI 5, pp. 461–462)

23: **A.** Nitroglycerin is most often prescribed as treatment of angina pectoris. (ECTSI 5, p. 450)

24: **C.** Supplemental oxygen must be given carefully to a patient who has COPD because a rapid rise in arterial oxygen may shut down the oxygen drive and eventually cause respiratory arrest. (ECTSI 5, p. 475)

25: **C.** Blockage in the coronary artery causes myocardial infarction. Oxygenated blood cannot reach the heart muscle and tissue dies. (ECTSI 5, p. 450)

26: **C.** Nitroglycerin acts to relieve cardiac pain by dilating the coronary arteries, allowing more oxygenated blood to reach the heart. (ECTSI 5, p. 450)

27: **A.** A patient who is going into insulin shock, but still conscious, should be given sips of fruit juice. (ECTSI 5, p. 488)

28: **B.** Insulin causes blood sugar (glucose) to be able to enter the cells in the body. (ECTSI 5, p. 483)

29: **B.** The principal physiologic difference between type I and type II diabetes is that with type I diabetes, a person does not produce adequate insulin. With type II diabetes, a person produces insulin, but the insulin's capacity to function is impaired. (ECTSI 5, p. 482)

30: **C.** The two most important questions to ask a conscious patient who is experiencing a diabetic emergency are as follows: "Have you taken insulin today?" and "Have you eaten today?" These questions can help you determine the type of diabetes the patient has and then how best to care for the patient. (ECTSI 5, p. 487)

31: **D.** An altered level of consciousness makes the patient's airway vulnerable. In this situation, you should provide prompt transport to the hospital, and give the patient nothing by mouth. (ECTSI 5, p. 488)

32: **B.** Insulin shock is caused by an excess amount of insulin due to any of the factors listed. (ECTSI 5, p. 486)

33: **B.** Sweet, fruity breath odor is a common sign of diabetic ketoacidosis. (ECTSI 5, p. 485)

34: **B.** Giving supplemental oxygen is the only appropriate treatment listed. (ECTSI 5, p. 477)

General Medical Emergencies

35: **C.** A spontaneous pneumothorax is best described as a rupture of the lung that allows air into the pleural space. (ECTSI 5, p. 471)

36: **D.** Large amounts of oxygen given at a high flow rate should not be given to a patient with emphysema. High levels of arterial oxygen can abolish the respiratory oxygen drive while the carbon dioxide level remains high. If the patient is depending on a low oxygen level to sustain breathing, the rapid rise might abolish this stimulus and cause respiratory arrest. (ECTSI 5, p. 475)

37: **D.** A patient with asthma may have an emergency epinephrine kit available. You may help the patient by finding the kit and assisting with administration. (ECTSI 5, p. 477)

38: **A.** Spasm and constriction of the bronchial tubes, resulting in congestion and difficulty in breathing is a physiologic description of asthma. (ECTSI 5, p. 472)

39: **C.** Of the conditions listed, emphysema is not considered a communicable disease. (ECTSI 5, p. 520)

40: **D.** Proper disposal of sharps consists of placing them in a puncture-resistant container without recapping, rinsing, or cutting. (ECTSI 5, p. 517)

41: **D.** Transmission of tuberculosis most commonly occurs through direct contact with a coughing patient or the patient's sputum. (ECTSI 5, p. 518)

42: **D.** A PPD skin test is performed on EMTs prior to employment to check for exposure to tuberculosis. (ECTSI 5, p. 515)

43: **B.** Proper body substance isolation measures do not include rinsing and recapping needles before disposal. Proper disposal of sharps consists of placing them into a puncture-resistant container immediately after use. (ECTSI 5, p. 517)

44: **D.** Of the situations listed, direct contact with blood-contaminated surfaces, such as those in the back of the ambulance, without proper protection present the greatest risk. (ECTSI 5, p. 520)

45: **D.** Many people with special medical problems wear bracelets or necklaces indicating the nature of their problem, such as "diabetic" or "allergic to penicillin." (ECTSI 5, p. 486)

Chapter 16

46: **C.** In this situation, you should perform a thorough assessment and then transport. The fact that the patient appears intoxicated does not change your responsibility to provide care. (ECTSI 5, p. 543)

47: **B.** In caring for an unconscious patient, you should determine responsiveness or level of consciousness immediately after you check for an open airway. (ECTSI 5, p. 544)

Chapter 17

Pediatric Emergencies

Chapter Goals

The exercises in this chapter are designed to help the student to:

- describe the pediatric patient.

- explain basic life support measures for a child and an infant.

- identify specific pediatric emergencies.

- describe proper care for a variety of pediatric emergencies.

Chapter 17

Multiple-Choice Questions

Select the correct answer for each of the following questions. Each question has only *one* correct or best answer.

1. Which of the following is a viral condition that may cause airway obstruction due to swelling of the lining of the larynx?

    A. Croup

    B. Epiglottitis

    C. Bronchitis

    D. Laryngitis

2. The first 30 days after birth a child is considered:

    A. a young child.

    B. a fetus.

    C. an infant.

    D. a neonate.

3. A seizure that accompanies a high fever, is of short duration, and requires no special treatment beyond airway maintenance is called:

    A. an epileptic seizure.

    B. a grand mal seizure.

    C. a focal motor seizure.

    D. a febrile convulsion.

4. A child who is dehydrated must be given prompt transport to the hospital due to the possibility that which of the following conditions may develop?

    A. Gastroenteritis

    B. Meningitis

    C. Shock

    D. Appendicitis

Pediatric Emergencies

5. Which of the following is a bacterial infection that produces severe swelling of the flap of tissue protecting the opening of the larynx?

   A. Croup

   B. Meningitis

   C. Gastroenteritis

   D. Epiglottitis

6. The proper size of an oropharyngeal airway for an infant or a child is roughly equal to the distance from the:

   A. tip of the patient's nose to the mouth.

   B. corner of the patient's mouth to the earlobe.

   C. tip of the patient's middle finger to the first knuckle.

   D. tip of the patient's little finger to the first knuckle.

7. During transport of a child who has a partial airway obstruction, you should:

   A. observe and record the child's level of consciousness using the Apgar scale.

   B. continue attempts to remove the obstruction by hyperextending the child's neck.

   C. administer high-flow oxygen with the oxygen mask held a bit away from the child's face.

   D. administer high-flow oxygen with the oxygen mask placed tightly over the child's mouth and nose.

8. The total circulating blood volume in an average-size newborn is:

   A. 100 to 300 mL.

   B. 300 to 500 mL.

   C. 500 mL to 1 L.

   D. 1 to 2 L.

Chapter 17

9. Which of the following conditions is an infection of the membranes covering the brain and spinal cord?

    A. Meningitis

    B. Rubeola

    C. Rubella

    D. Gastroenteritis

10. You are called to a home in which you suspect a young child has been sexually abused. Your primary responsibility in this situation is to:

    A. ask the child to identify the abuser.

    B. conduct a thorough examination, including the genitalia.

    C. transport the child before he or she can wash, urinate, or defecate.

    D. report the situation and wait for law enforcement officials to arrive at the scene.

11. A 5-year-old child has ingested a poison, and the poison control center recommends that vomiting be induced. The child should be given:

    A. 2 tablespoons of dry mustard in a glass of water.

    B. 2 tablespoons of syrup of ipecac in a glass of water.

    C. 1 tablespoon of dry mustard in a glass of water.

    D. 1 tablespoon of syrup of ipecac in a glass of water.

12. A child has swallowed an unknown amount of Drano drain cleaner. Your care for the patient should consist of:

    A. providing prompt transport without inducing vomiting.

    B. sticking your finger down the child's throat to induce vomiting.

    C. giving the child 1 tablespoon of syrup of ipecac in a glass of water to induce vomiting.

    D. giving the child 1 tablespoon of dry mustard in a glass of water to induce vomiting.

Pediatric Emergencies

13. What is the best technique for providing artificial ventilation to a toddler who is not breathing?

    A. Supplemental oxygen using a bag-valve-mask

    B. Supplemental oxygen using a nasal cannula

    C. Mouth-to-mask resuscitation

    D. Supplemental oxygen using a demand valve resuscitator

14. What is the most serious cause of abdominal pain in childhood?

    A. Gastroenteritis

    B. Dehydration

    C. Appendicitis

    D. Gallbladder disease

15. The most dangerous fevers in children are those caused by:

    A. heatstroke.

    B. heat exhaustion.

    C. gastroenteritis.

    D. dehydration.

16. A child who is having an epileptic seizure begins to turn blue. You should first:

    A. place your fingers in the patient's mouth to move the tongue.

    B. attempt to pry the patient's jaw open using your fingers.

    C. wait until the seizure ends before doing anything.

    D. attempt to restore the airway.

Chapter 17

17. You are called to the scene of an automobile accident in which an unrestrained child has been thrown from the car. The child is unconscious and believed to have a spinal injury and a fractured leg. You should prepare to immobilize the child by:

    A. flexing the neck to open the airway and applying a child's size cervical collar.

    B. picking up the child using the front cradle and moving the child to the ambulance stretcher.

    C. securing the child to a backboard with the foot of the board slightly elevated.

    D. placing padding under the child's shoulders to prevent excessive neck flexion before securing the child to the backboard.

18. A child who has ingested an unknown poison is drifting in and out of consciousness. The proper course of action is to:

    A. give the child 1 tablespoon of syrup of ipecac in water.

    B. give the child 1 tablespoon of dry mustard in water.

    C. provide transport without attempting to induce vomiting.

    D. attempt to suction the mouth.

19. A child with a head injury should be transported to the hospital:

    A. on a backboard with the legs slightly elevated.

    B. on a backboard with the head slightly elevated.

    C. in a side-lying position to prevent aspiration of vomitus.

    D. cradled in your arms and supported by your shoulder.

20. Which of the following signs strongly suggests early stages of shock?

    A. Systolic blood pressure of less than 50 mm Hg

    B. Diastolic blood pressure of less than 50 mm Hg

    C. A combined blood pressure of less than 100 mm Hg

    D. Delayed capillary refill time

Pediatric Emergencies

21. A child in shock should not be given anything to eat or drink because the:

    A. airway may become obstructed.

    B. child may have an allergic reaction.

    C. shock may reverse itself before the child is examined by a physician.

    D. child's stomach must be empty in the event that surgery is necessary.

22. A child with a severe soft tissue injury to the leg has rather extensive bleeding, which has frightened the child. The best way to control the bleeding in this situation is to apply:

    A. a conventional tourniquet.

    B. pressure to the femoral artery.

    C. direct pressure with a dry, sterile dressing.

    D. a blood pressure cuff to act as a tourniquet.

23. What is the single most important assessment finding to obtain in a child who has a head injury?

    A. The difference between the systolic and diastolic blood pressures

    B. A baseline level of consciousness and any changes

    C. A series of blood pressure readings

    D. The pulse rate

24. Before applying a splint or aligning an injured extremity on a child, you should:

    A. elevate the extremity.

    B. take a blood pressure reading on that extremity.

    C. ask the child to bend the extremity.

    D. assess distal neurovascular function.

Chapter 17

25. Assessment of distal neurovascular function includes assessments of capillary refill time and motor function, along with evaluations of:

   A. blood pressure and pulse.

   B. sensation and pulse.

   C. sensation and skin color.

   D. sensation and flexibility.

Answers

1: **A.** Croup is a viral condition that may cause airway obstruction in children due to swelling of the lining of the larynx below its opening. (ECTSI 5, pp. 561–562)

2: **D.** The first 30 days after birth a child is considered a neonate. (ECTSI 5, p. 556)

3: **D.** A febrile convulsion is a seizure that occurs in some children, accompanying a high fever. (ECTSI 5, p. 566)

4: **C.** A child who is dehydrated must be given prompt transport to the hospital due to the possibility that shock will develop. (ECTSI 5, pp. 566–567)

5: **D.** Epiglottitis is a bacterial infection that produces severe swelling of the epiglottis, the flap of tissue protecting the opening to the larynx. (ECTSI 5, p. 562)

6: **B.** The distance from the corner of the patient's mouth to the earlobe is the proper size for an oropharyngeal airway for an infant or child. (ECTSI 5, p. 562)

7: **C.** While transporting a child with a partial airway obstruction to the hospital, you should administer high-flow oxygen by placing the oxygen mask gently over the child's mouth and nose and holding it a bit away from the face. (ECTSI 5, p. 560)

8: **B.** The total circulating blood volume in an average-size newborn is 300 to 500 mL. (ECTSI 5, p. 564)

9: **A.** Meningitis is an extremely serious viral or bacterial infection that affects the membranes covering the brain and spinal cord. (ECTSI 5, p. 566)

Pediatric Emergencies

10: **C.** If sexual abuse of a child is suspected, the child should not be allowed to wash, urinate, or defecate before being examined by a physician. You are not responsible for making judgments about the potential abuser. Your state will have established protocols concerning your reporting responsibilities. (ECTSI 5, p. 569)

11: **D.** A 5-year-old child who is awake and alert should be given 1 tablespoon of syrup of ipecac in a glass of water if a poison has been ingested and the poison control center recommends that vomiting be induced. (ECTSI 5, p. 567)

12: **A.** If a child has swallowed a strong acid, alkali (such as Drano drain cleaner), or a petroleum product, vomiting should not be induced. (ECTSI 5, p. 567)

13: **C.** Mouth-to-mask resuscitation is the preferred technique of artificial ventilation, particularly if the child is large enough so that a tight seal cannot be made over both the nose and mouth together. (ECTSI 5, p. 125)

14: **C.** Appendicitis is the most serious cause of abdominal pain in children. (ECTSI 5, p. 566)

15: **A.** Of the conditions listed, heatstroke is the most dangerous cause of fever in a child. (ECTSI 5, p. 566)

16: **D.** When a child who is having an epileptic seizure becomes cyanotic, you must attempt to restore the airway. Gentle extension of the neck will open the airway partially. Ventilations through the nose in a patient with clenched teeth should be facilitated by keeping the nasal passages clear with suction. (ECTSI 5, p. 566)

17: **D.** You should assume that any unconscious child who has been involved in an accident has a spinal injury. As you prepare to immobilize the patient, you should avoid flexing the neck or back. Before securing the child to a backboard, you should place padding under the child's shoulders to compensate for the child's disproportionately larger head size. (ECTSI 5, p. 564)

18: **C.** Vomiting should not be induced in an unconscious or partially conscious child who has ingested a poison. (ECTSI 5, p. 567)

19: **B.** A child with a head injury should be secured to a backboard and transported to the hospital with the head of the backboard slightly elevated. (ECTSI 5, p. 564)

Chapter 17

20: **D.** Delayed capillary refill time in a peripheral extremity strongly suggests early stages of shock in a child. (ECTSI 5, p. 564)

21: **D.** A child in shock should not be given anything to eat or drink because the stomach must be empty in the event that surgery is needed. (ECTSI 5, p. 564)

22: **C.** The best way to control bleeding in an extremity injury to a child is to apply direct pressure with a dry, sterile dressing. (ECTSI 5, p. 565)

23: **B.** A baseline assessment of level of consciousness, followed by periodic reassessment, is considered the single most important clinical finding to obtain in a child who has a head injury. (ECTSI 5, pp. 564–565)

24: **D.** Before applying a splint or aligning an injured extremity on a child, you should assess distal neurovascular function. (ECTSI 5, p. 565)

25: **B.** Assessment of the distal neurovascular function includes checking the pulse, capillary refill time, sensation, and motor function. (ECTSI 5, p. 565)

Chapter 18

Substance Abuse

> ### *Chapter Goals*

The exercises in this chapter are designed to help the student to:

- identify effects of alcohol on the body.

- describe appropriate treatment of injuries and/or illnesses that result from alchohol abuse.

- list several types of drugs commonly abused, their routes of administration, and their common effects on the body.

- describe appropriate treatment of injuries and/or illnesses that result from drug overdose and abuse.

- list the signs and symptoms of drug withdrawal.

Chapter 18

Multiple-Choice Questions

Select the correct answer for each of the following questions. Each question has only *one* correct or best answer.

1. You are called to the apartment of an 18-year-old man who has reportedly taken "some drugs." The patient is depressed, sluggish, has slurred speech, and lacks coordination. These signs and symptoms suggest an overdose of:

    A. cocaine.

    B. barbiturates.

    C. amphetamines.

    D. hallucinogens.

2. A woman who has consumed a large quantity of alcohol begins coughing and vomiting. Her respirations are deep and somewhat labored. At first, the vomitus is clear to light yellow, but then it turns reddish brown. The patient is uncooperative and states that "this is all his fault" as she points toward a man sitting nearby. He states that he is the husband and that "she always does this." Your care of this patient should include giving:

    A. the patient coffee to "sober her up" before transport.

    B. instructions to the husband to "sober her up" and referring the couple to counseling.

    C. the patient plenty of water to drink and then providing transport.

    D. supplemental oxygen and then providing transport in a side-lying position.

3. A patient with delirium tremens (DTs) is experiencing a seizure upon your arrival. Treatment of this type of seizure should include:

    A. "sobering up" the patient.

    B. restraining the patient, using a bite stick if necessary.

    C. protecting the patient from self-injury and giving oxygen, if necessary.

    D. securing the patient to a long backboard, giving oxygen, and providing immediate transport.

Substance Abuse

4. A patient with DTs can go into shock due to:

   A. convulsions.

   B. hallucinations.

   C. high blood levels of alcohol.

   D. fluid loss due to fever, sweating, and vomiting.

5. What is the principal effect of alcohol, tranquilizers, barbiturates, and narcotics?

   A. They depress the CNS.

   B. They cause hallucinations.

   C. They are considered "uppers."

   D. They dehydrate the body, but present no immediate threat to life.

6. You are called to the home of a 42-year-old man who appears incoherent and is throwing objects at mirrors and windows. He says, "the cat is following me," and that he "needs to jump." You should report to medical control that the patient has likely taken:

   A. a barbiturate.

   B. a stimulant.

   C. a hallucinogen.

   D. heroin.

7. You are called to the city park where a teenager is found lying on a park bench mumbling incoherently, holding a half-full bottle of cheap wine. The patient appears very groggy and cannot sit up, but he appears to have no injuries. The patient has warm, dry skin, a fruity breath odor, and dried vomit on his clothing. Your first step in caring for this patient should be to:

   A. call his parents to pick him up.

   B. give oxygen, if necessary, and provide immediate transport.

   C. give the patient plenty of water to drink and offer to drive him home.

   D. perform a thorough assessment, then offer to drive him home if he is not injured.

Chapter 18

8. A pregnant 33-year-old woman is having contractions 1 minute apart when you arrive at her home. She is screaming for you to "Get it out! Get it out!" as you walk into the bedroom. As you prepare for an emergency home delivery, you notice a strong smell of alcohol in the room. As the baby is born, it appears smaller than full term and smells of alcohol. Immediately after delivery, you should:

   A. monitor the baby's respirations and provide immediate transport for both mother and baby.

   B. ask the mother how much she had been drinking before delivery and why she would harm her baby that way.

   C. call the appropriate social services agency to report the situation and then transport the mother and baby to the hospital.

   D. prepare the mother and baby for transport and collect any liquor bottles you can find for evidence of alcohol abuse.

9. Which of the following substances may be used legally, in certain circumstances, in the United States?

   A. Heroin

   B. Phencyclidine

   C. Crack

   D. Morphine

10. In most states, a person is considered legally intoxicated if his or her blood alcohol level is:

    A. 0.04%.

    B. 0.06%.

    C. 0.08%.

    D. 0.10%.

Substance Abuse

11. You are sent to the home of a young couple where a woman meets you at the door. She tells you her husband is "drunk again" and that she is tired of his "partying." You find her husband sitting on their bed, quietly watching television. His eyes are glassy, he smells of alcohol, and he is slowly opening and closing a switchblade. He does not respond to any of your questions. Your first step in handling this situation is to:

    A. tell the woman because her husband is not sick or injured, this is a matter for the police and then leave.

    B. call law enforcement officials and then wait for them to arrive before you do anything.

    C. try to convince the patient to give you the knife so you can perform a thorough examination.

    D. begin your primary and secondary assessments, and gently take away the knife as you take the patient's pulse.

12. The result of tolerance to a certain drug is that the user must:

    A. use extremely large doses to achieve the desired effect.

    B. use extremely small doses or risk an allergic reaction.

    C. avoid using the drug altogether or risk cardiac arrest.

    D. change the route of administration to achieve the desired effect.

13. Widely dilated pupils are characteristic of an overdose of:

    A. heroin.

    B. morphine.

    C. cocaine.

    D. barbiturates.

14. A patient with DTs has been vomiting and is sweaty and shaky. You should prepare for transport by placing the patient on the ambulance stretcher with the:

    A. patient in a sitting position.

    B. feet elevated, and the head turned to the side.

    C. head elevated, and the head turned to the side.

    D. knees bent, and the patient in a side-lying position.

Chapter 18

15. Codeine is considered:

    A. a barbiturate.

    B. a stimulant.

    C. an opium compound.

    D. a hypnotic compound.

16. Treatment of a patient who has taken an overdose of barbiturates should focus on ensuring that:

    A. vomiting is induced and collected prior to transport.

    B. the patient understands that he or she has a drug problem.

    C. the airway is clear, respirations are supported, and transport provided.

    D. the airway is clear, the patient is restrained, if necessary, and transport provided.

17. Severe hypoxia is commonly associated with an overdose of which of the following substances?

    A. Crack

    B. Alcohol

    C. Aerosol fumes

    D. Anabolic steroids

18. You are called to the home of a teenage girl who has pierced her left eye with a pencil in what her mother says was an attempt to "stop the bugs from crawling in." The eye is bleeding and the pencil is impaled in the sclera. The patient is anxious, agitated, and in a great deal of pain. In this situation, the impaled object should be:

    A. removed, and the patient reassured that the bugs are gone.

    B. removed, and the wound covered with a dry, sterile dressing.

    C. stabilized in place with a roller bandage and secured with a dry, sterile dressing.

    D. cleansed thoroughly with sterile saline solution, stabilized in place with a roller bandage and then secured with a dry, sterile dressing.

Substance Abuse

Answers

1: **B.** These signs and symptoms suggest an overdose of barbiturates. (ECTSI 5, p. 528)

2: **D.** The patient's signs and symptoms indicate that the large quantity of alcohol consumed and subsequent vomiting have possibly irritated the esophagus and stomach. Hematemesis, blood in the vomitus, can occur when the lining of the esophagus is lacerated by repeated forceful vomiting. The patient is also experiencing some difficulty breathing. Appropriate care would include giving supplemental oxygen and then providing transport. The patient should be transported in a side-lying position due to the potential for more vomiting. (ECTSI 5, p. 526)

3: **C.** Seizures that accompany delirium tremens should be treated like any other seizures. The patient should not be restrained or secured to a backboard during the seizure, although adequate protection must be provided to prevent self-injury. Oxygen should be given, and the patient monitored for vomiting. (ECTSI 5, p. 527)

4: **D.** The loss of fluids due to sweating, fever, and vomiting can cause a patient to go into shock. (ECTSI 5, p. 527)

5: **A.** All of these substances act to depress the central nervous system (CNS). (ECTSI 5, pp. 526–528)

6: **C.** These findings suggest that the patient has taken a hallucinogen. (ECTSI 5, pp. 533–534)

7: **B.** The patient's signs and symptoms suggest a possible impending diabetic coma. Occasionally, patients with diabetes are mistakenly identified as intoxicated, even in circumstances similar to this patient. The warm, dry skin and fruity breath odor should alert you to the possibility of a diabetic, not substance abuse, emergency. (ECTSI 5, pp. 485–486)

8: **A.** Your appropriate course of action would be to carry out the delivery as best you can, monitor the baby's respirations, and transport both mother and baby immediately. Do not judge or lecture the mother; just help with the delivery and get both the baby and the mother to the hospital. (ECTSI 5, pp. 590–591)

9: **D.** Of the substances listed, only morphine is considered an exempt narcotic; the other substances are regarded as absolutely illegal in the United States. (ECTSI 5, p. 528)

Chapter 18

10: **D.** While it may vary somewhat from state to state, in most states a person is considered legally intoxicated with a blood alcohol level of 0.10%. This percentage means that 0.1 gram of alcohol exists in each 100 mL of circulating blood. (ECTSI 5, p. 527)

11: **B.** The first step in handling a situation in which a patient is armed is to call law enforcement officials and wait until they arrive before you do anything. Your priority is to protect yourself and the patient. Do not take your eyes off the patient and be alert for any obviously aggressive behavior. Do not try to disarm the patient yourself. This is a job for law enforcement officials. Also, it is not appropriate to leave the scene, as the patient may injure himself or his wife. (ECTSI 5, pp. 652–653)

12. **A.** The result of tolerance to a certain drug is that the user must use extremely large doses to achieve the desired effect. During a period when the drug is not used, tolerance is often lost as rapidly as it developed. (ECTSI 5, pp. 535–536)

13. **D.** Widely dilated pupils are characteristic of an overdose of barbiturates. (ECTSI 5, p. 549)

14. **B.** You should prepare to transport this patient by placing him on the ambulance stretcher with the feet elevated and the head turned to the side to prevent aspiration if there is more vomiting. (ECTSI 5, p. 527)

15: **C.** Codeine is considered an opium compound. (ECTSI 5, p. 527)

16: **C.** In general, treatment of a patient who has taken an overdose of barbiturates should focus on ensuring that the airway is clear, respirations are supported, and transport provided. Today, with increasingly common multi-drug use, the clinical picture of the patient may not be as clear. Therefore, you should also assess for additional injuries or illness that might make full life support mandatory. (ECTSI 5, p. 530)

17: **C.** Severe hypoxia is commonly associated with an overdose of an inhalant, such as fumes from an aerosol can, or those in a bottle of glue or a can of gasoline. The hypoxia is often caused by the device, usually of makeshift construction, that is used to inhale the active vapors. Frequently, the substances are inhaled from within a closed plastic bag that collapses and obstructs the airway. (ECTSI 5, p. 538)

Substance Abuse

18: **C.** In this situation, the patient has injured herself, perhaps as a result of taking a hallucinogen or as a result of some type of withdrawal. Regardless of the cause, the patient's eye injury needs to be addressed. Objects impaled in the eye must be removed by the physician; therefore, the pencil must be stabilized with a roller bandage and secured in place. In the event that the patient becomes combative, you may need to restrain her to protect the eye. (ECTSI 5, pp. 354, 534)

Chapter 19

Childbirth

Chapter Goals

The exercises in this chapter are designed to help the student to:

- identify the early signs of labor.

- describe the three stages of labor.

- describe the steps of a normal delivery.

- describe various abnormal deliveries.

- list the proper steps in caring for a newborn.

Childbirth

Multiple-Choice Questions

Select the correct answer for each of the following questions. Each question has only *one* correct or best answer.

1. A woman who is pregnant for the first time is having contractions every 5 minutes. In this situation, you should:

    A. prepare for an emergency delivery.

    B. transport the woman to the hospital.

    C. help the woman to walk around between contractions.

    D. hold the woman's legs together to slow down delivery.

2. A newborn is not breathing on its own shortly after delivery. The 1-minute Apgar score is 4. The first step in caring for the newborn is to:

    A. stimulate the newborn by gently shaking.

    B. resuction the nose and mouth.

    C. wrap the newborn in warm blankets.

    D. begin CPR.

3. A baby who weighs less than 5 1/2 lb at birth is considered:

    A. immature.

    B. premature.

    C. full-term.

    D. normal.

Chapter 19

4. A woman who is having her third baby tells you she must move her bowels. The most appropriate step would be to:

   A. provide prompt transport because there is still plenty of time before the delivery.

   B. ask her if she is about to deliver, and if she says no, provide prompt transport.

   C. provide immediate transport because it is always safer to deliver at the hospital.

   D. prepare to deliver the baby at the scene, because delivery is about to occur.

5. If a woman's abdomen remains unusually large after delivery, you should prepare for:

   A. a multiple birth.

   B. severe bleeding.

   C. a delay in delivery of the placenta.

   D. partial delivery of the placenta.

6. If a woman is having her first child, labor will probably:

   A. last several days.

   B. last about 7 hours.

   C. be longer than for a woman who has had other children.

   D. be shorter than for a woman who has had other children.

7. You note excessive bleeding from the vagina following the normal delivery of a newborn. Before transport, you should:

   A. press the uterus toward the vagina.

   B. pack the vagina with sterile, absorbent material.

   C. allow the woman to sit up and drink small amounts of water.

   D. massage the uterus, place the woman in the shock position, and give oxygen.

Childbirth

8. A woman in labor appears to have a part of the umbilical cord protruding from the vagina. You should first place the woman in a shock position, and then carefully:

    A. push the cord back into the vagina and provide prompt transport.

    B. insert your gloved finger into the vagina and gently push the baby's head away from the umbilical cord.

    C. push the baby's head back into the vagina and provide prompt transport.

    D. moisten the cord with sterile saline solution and provide prompt transport.

9. A woman who is having her first child is having contractions 2 minutes apart. You should:

    A. prepare to deliver the baby at the scene.

    B. provide slow transport while monitoring the woman's vital signs.

    C. examine for crowning before deciding whether to transport.

    D. place the woman in a shock position and provide immediate transport.

10. As you prepare to assist a woman in labor, you should ask whether this is her first child, because:

    A. labor may be longer if it is the first birth.

    B. labor may be shorter if it is the first birth.

    C. labor may be longer if there were previous births.

    D. the hospital will need this information for its state records.

11. You are assisting at an emergency home delivery, and the baby's head is delivered still covered by the membranes of the unruptured sac. The next step is to:

    A. wait for the sac to break on its own, then clear the baby's nose and mouth.

    B. leave the sac intact, monitor the baby's vital signs, and provide immediate transport.

    C. wait until the delivery is complete, carefully puncture the sac with your gloved fingers, a sterile clamp, or scissors, and clear the baby's nose and mouth.

    D. immediately, but carefully, puncture the sac with your gloved fingers, a sterile clamp, or scissors, and clear the baby's nose and mouth.

Chapter 19

12. You should support delivery of the baby's head by:

    A. placing your hand over the head as it emerges and placing very gentle pressure on it.

    B. placing one hand at the top of the head and the other in back.

    C. maintaining finger pressure against the center of the baby's skull.

    D. placing the palm of your hand firmly against the back of the baby's skull.

13. What five areas of activity in the newborn are evaluated by the Apgar score?

    A. Cardiac rate, eye tracking, muscle tone, color, strength of cry

    B. Cardiac rate, respiratory effort, muscle tone, reflex irritability, color

    C. Grip strength, respiratory effort, muscle tone, color, strength of cry

    D. Grip strength, eye tracking, respiratory effort, muscle tone, color

14. Immediately following delivery of the head, you must:

    A. apply gentle pressure over the woman's abdomen.

    B. check the position of the umbilical cord.

    C. check the woman for bleeding.

    D. suction the baby's nose and mouth.

15. The fetus develops inside the:

    A. umbilicus.

    B. placenta.

    C. fundus.

    D. uterus.

16. The fluid-filled, bag-like membrane in which the fetus grows is called the:

    A. uterine sac.

    B. perineal sac.

    C. amniotic sac.

    D. placental sac.

Childbirth

17. During a normal delivery, the baby's head is usually tilted:

    A. chin down.

    B. posteriorly, facedown.

    C. posteriorly, to one side.

    D. anteriorly, with the chin up.

18. Delivery of the head during a breech birth must occur within how many minutes to prevent suffocation?

    A. 4

    B. 3

    C. 2

    D. 1

19. The developing fetus receives nourishment from the mother through the:

    A. placenta.

    B. amniotic fluid.

    C. uterus.

    D. vagina.

20. During an emergency home delivery, you should place the woman:

    A. on the floor with a clean sheet under her buttocks.

    B. on a bed with a clean sheet under her buttocks.

    C. in a comfortable chair covered with a sterile towel.

    D. on a sturdy table covered with a sterile towel.

21. A prolapsed umbilical cord is dangerous because:

    A. the cord may be wrapped around the baby's neck, causing strangulation.

    B. the baby's head may tear the cord, causing hemorrhage.

    C. the baby's head may compress the cord, cutting off all circulation.

    D. the cord may pull the placenta free during delivery.

Chapter 19

22. You see the baby's arm rather than the head as the woman says she needs to push. The most appropriate course of action would be to:

    A. try to gently push the arm back into the vagina.

    B. cover the arm with a sterile towel and provide immediate transport.

    C. place the woman on her back and gently press her abdomen.

    D. insert your gloved fingers into the vagina and gently try to turn the baby.

23. After the placenta has been delivered, it should be saved and transported to the hospital so that hospital staff can determine if:

    A. it has been completely expelled.

    B. its weight needs to be recorded for legal purposes.

    C. its shape suggests hidden deformities in the newborn.

    D. its blood could be used if the newborn needs a transfusion.

24. Your care of a premature baby should include:

    A. keeping the baby cool.

    B. removing the clamp on the umbilical cord.

    C. keeping the mouth and nose clear of mucus.

    D. directing a stream of oxygen directly into the baby's mouth.

25. During what stage of labor would you assist with delivery of the placenta?

    A. First

    B. Second

    C. Third

    D. Fourth

Childbirth

Answers

1: **B.** A woman having contractions 5 minutes apart should be transported to the hospital. (ECTSI 5, p. 577)

2: **B.** The first step in caring for an infant who is not breathing spontaneously after 30 seconds is to resuction the nose and mouth. (ECTSI 5, p. 586)

3: **B.** A premature baby is one who delivers before 8 months gestation or weighs less than 5 1/2 lb at birth. (ECTSI 5, p. 591)

4: **D.** If a woman who has had a child tells you she feels as if she must move her bowels, you should prepare to deliver the baby at the scene. The baby's head is pressing on her rectum and delivery is about to occur. (ECTSI 5, p. 577)

5: **A.** A multiple birth should be suspected if the woman's abdomen remains unusually large after the baby is born. (ECTSI 5, p. 590)

6: **C.** Labor varies with each person, but it generally lasts longer in a situation where the first child is being born. (ECTSI 5, p. 577)

7: **D.** A woman who has excessive vaginal bleeding following a normal delivery should have first a sanitary pad placed over the vagina to begin controlling the bleeding. You should massage her uterus, then place her in the shock position, administer oxygen, monitor vital signs, and then provide transport to the hospital. (ECTSI 5, p. 585)

8: **B.** When presented with a prolapsed umbilical cord, you should place the woman in the shock position, carefully insert your gloved finger into the vagina, and then gently push the baby's head away from the umbilical cord. (ECTSI 5, pp. 588–589)

9: **C.** A woman expecting her first child is having contractions 2 minutes apart. You should examine for crowning before deciding whether there is time to transport. (ECTSI 5, p. 577)

10: **A.** It is important to ask a woman in labor whether this is her first child, because labor may be longer if it is a first birth. (ECTSI 5, p. 577)

11: **D.** If the baby's head is still covered by the membranes of the amniotic sac after delivery, you must break the membranes immediately to prevent suffocation. You should then clear the baby's nose and mouth, and then complete the delivery. (ECTSI 5, pp. 585–586)

Chapter 19

12: **A.** Support the delivery of the baby's head by placing your hand over the head as it emerges and then exert very gentle pressure. However, avoid pressing your fingers into the baby's fontanelles. (ECTSI 5, p. 580)

13: **B.** The five areas of activity evaluated by the Apgar score are cardiac rate, respiratory effort, muscle tone, reflex irritability, and color. (ECTSI 5, p. 584)

14: **B.** Immediately following delivery of the head, you must check the position of the umbilical cord to make sure it is not wrapped around the baby's neck. (ECTSI 5, p. 580)

15: **D.** The fetus develops within the uterus. (ECTSI 5, p. 575)

16: **C.** The fetus grows inside the fluid-filled bag-like amniotic sac. (ECTSI 5, p. 576)

17: **C.** During a normal delivery, the baby's head is usually tilted to one side. (ECTSI 5, p. 580)

18: **B.** With a breech delivery, the baby's head should deliver within 3 minutes. If it does not, provide rapid transport while holding the baby's airway open to prevent suffocation. (ECTSI 5, p. 588)

19: **A.** The growing fetus receives nourishment from the woman through the placenta. (ECTSI 5, pp. 575–576)

20: **D.** In an emergency home delivery, the woman should be placed on a sturdy table, if possible, covered with a sterile towel. (ECTSI 5, p. 579)

21: **C.** Prolapse of the umbilical cord is very dangerous because the baby's head may compress the cord, cutting off all circulation. (ECTSI 5, pp. 588–589)

22: **B.** If you are confronted with a limb presentation, cover the limb with a sterile towel and provide immediate transport because this type of delivery must take place in the hospital. (ECTSI 5, p. 588)

23: **A.** The hospital staff needs to examine the placenta after delivery to make sure that it has been completely expelled. (ECTSI 5, p. 585)

24: **C.** Your care of a premature baby should include keeping the mouth and nose clear of mucus. (ECTSI 5, p. 592)

25: **C.** Delivery of the placenta occurs in the third stage of labor. (ECTSI 5, p. 584)

Chapter 20

Environmental Injuries

Chapter Goals

The exercises in this chapter are designed to help the student to:

- identify the different layers and functions of the skin.

- describe the various degrees of burns, their appearance, and severity.

- explain how the Rule of Nines is used to assess the severity of burns.

- explain proper emergency care for various types of burns.

- describe the risks of exposure to various hazardous materials.

- describe the three forms of heat exposure.

- explain the importance of self-protection against cold or heat exposure.

- discuss the mechanisms of drowning and near drowning.

- explain proper emergency care measures for near-drowning victims.

Chapter 20

Multiple-Choice Questions

Select the correct answer for each of the following questions. Each question has only *one* correct or best answer.

1. Carbon monoxide is a colorless, odorless gas that:

   A. destroys white blood cells.

   B. prevents blood from clotting.

   C. paralyzes the respiratory system.

   D. blocks the transport of oxygen to body tissues.

2. The goals of treatment of hypothermia in the field are to:

   A. rewarm the patient and prevent shock.

   B. rewarm the patient and prevent blood loss.

   C. stabilize the vital signs and rewarm the patient.

   D. stabilize the vital signs and prevent further heat loss.

3. Which of the following is considered the most dangerous type of ionizing radiation due to its ability to penetrate the human body?

   A. Alpha rays

   B. Beta rays

   C. Gamma rays

   D. Energy rays

4. Accidental contact or ingestion resulting in absorption into the bloodstream is the greatest danger associated with what type of ionizing radiation?

   A. Alpha rays

   B. Beta rays

   C. Gamma rays

   D. Energy rays

Environmental Injuries

5. A man is injured in an industrial accident in which he is also exposed to radiation. The source of radiation is still present. You should first put on appropriate protective clothing and then:

    A. begin assessment without moving the patient.

    B. remove the patient's clothes and place them in a container.

    C. rapidly move the patient away from the radiation source.

    D. give supplemental oxygen.

6. A woman has third-degree burns on her arms and chest as a result of a house fire. You should stop any further burning by:

    A. immersing the burning skin in cool water for no more than 10 minutes.

    B. wrapping the burned areas with sterile, saline-moistened pressure dressings.

    C. placing the patient on a bed of ice for 30 minutes.

    D. applying cooling lotions to the burned areas.

7. The Rule of Nines is modified for an infant because:

    A. infants get severely burned.

    B. infants are smaller than adults.

    C. there is less surface area to be affected.

    D. more area is taken up by the infant's head and less by the legs.

8. What is the greatest danger to a patient who has sustained a burn?

    A. Shock

    B. Infection

    C. Air embolism

    D. Respiratory problems

Chapter 20

9. Shivering in the presence of hypothermia indicates that the:

    A. musculoskeletal system is damaged.

    B. nerve endings are damaged, causing loss of muscle control.

    C. body is trying to generate more heat through muscular activity.

    D. circulatory system is impaired, and the body cannot maintain its temperature.

10. Emergency treatment of heatstroke is focused primarily on:

    A. decreasing the patient's body temperature.

    B. replacing salt lost through sweating.

    C. restoring normal breathing.

    D. preventing convulsions.

11. A patient who has hypothermia has lost the ability to:

    A. protect the body against windchill.

    B. keep blood sugar (glucose) at safe levels.

    C. fight infection.

    D. generate body heat.

12. The best way to ease the pain of burns to the eye caused by a light source is to:

    A. cover each eye with dry dressings and paper cones or cups.

    B. cover each eye with sterile, moist pads and an eye shield.

    C. flush each eye with sterile water or saline solution.

    D. gently massage the injured eyelid.

13. Emergency treatment of an air embolism should include providing basic life support measures and then:

    A. providing transport to the nearest recompression chamber.

    B. giving the patient salt tablets and plenty of water to drink.

    C. applying hot packs and providing immediate transport to the hospital.

    D. helping the patient walk around to maintain circulation.

Environmental Injuries

14. You arrive at the home of a 13-year-old girl who is floating facedown in the swimming pool. Her mother is at the side of the pool screaming "Do something!" You and your partner should put on PFDs, jump in the pool, and then:

    A. rotate the upper half of her body as a unit until she is faceup.

    B. rotate her entire body as a unit and pull her out of the pool.

    C. turn her head to the side and begin rescue breathing.

    D. turn her head to the side and give four back blows.

15. Which of the following conditions may develop as a result of severe hypothermia?

    A. Cardiac thrombosis

    B. Cardiac arrhythmia

    C. Congestive heart failure

    D. Cerebrovascular accident

16. The amount of ionizing radiation exposure that a person receives depends on the:

    A. age of the person.

    B. body size of the person.

    C. general health of the person.

    D. distance of the person from the radiation source.

17. A teenage boy is successfully resuscitated at the scene after a near-drowning accident. Your next step in caring for the patient is to:

    A. advise him to visit his own doctor as soon as possible.

    B. provide transport to the hospital.

    C. provide transport to the patient's doctor.

    D. take the patient home.

American Academy of Orthopaedic Surgeons

Chapter 20

18. A man is weak and dizzy, has a headache, and shows early signs of shock after sitting in the sun for 2 hours. Your care of this patient should begin with:

    A. moving him to a cool area, treating him for shock, and giving him water to drink.

    B. moving him to a cool area, treating him for shock, and giving him salt tablets mixed in water to drink.

    C. moving him into a cool area, advising him to rest any cramping muscles, and giving him a diluted balanced electrolyte solution to drink.

    D. moving him into an air conditioned ambulance, covering him with wet towels or sheets, and providing immediate transport.

19. A man who has been exposed to a hot, humid climate for a long period of time has very hot, dry, slightly red skin. His armpits are dry, and his body temperature is 104°F. He states that he feels ill. These signs and symptoms suggest:

    A. heat collapse.

    B. heatstroke.

    C. heat cramps.

    D. heat exhaustion.

20. The principal goal in emergency treatment of heat exposure is to:

    A. provide rapid transport.

    B. make the patient comfortable.

    C. replace lost fluids with salt water.

    D. reduce the patient's body temperature.

21. You are called to the home of a woman who has frostbite. Upon arrival, you find that she is in her warm house, but there is a snowstorm beginning outside. The nearest hospital is 1 hour away. In this situation, treatment should consist of:

    A. rubbing the affected area with snow.

    B. rubbing the affected area with your warm hand.

    C. immersing the affected area in a warm water bath.

    D. immersing the affected area in an ice water bath.

Environmental Injuries

22. A 3-year-old child is found at the bottom of an ice-covered pond after being submerged for about 15 minutes. The patient is not breathing and has no palpable pulse. The most appropriate course of action would be to:

   A. pronounce the child dead.

   B. clear the airway and begin CPR.

   C. give supplemental oxygen and begin rewarming.

   D. wrap the child in blankets and give back blows.

23. Hypothermia can be defined as:

   A. progressive heating of the body.

   B. progressive cooling of the body.

   C. progressive fluid loss through sweating.

   D. progressively worse circulation in the extremities.

24. Treatment of hypothermia at the scene should include:

   A. rewarming the patient in an ambulance heated to 95°F.

   B. immersion in water at a temperature of between 100° to 112°F.

   C. preventing further heat loss by removing the patient from the cold environment.

   D. rewarming the patient with hot packs, heated blankets, and warm, wet head wraps.

25. The condition that occurs when the skin freezes, but deeper tissues do not, is called:

   A. immersion foot.

   B. hypothermia.

   C. frostbite.

   D. frostnip.

Chapter 20

26. A woman has frostbite in both feet after walking several miles in a frozen field. Her feet are white, hard, and cold to touch. Treatment at the scene should include:

    A. removing her wet clothing and covering her feet with dry, sterile dressings.

    B. removing her wet clothing and rubbing her feet briskly with a warm, wet cloth.

    C. trying to restore circulation by helping her walk around.

    D. rubbing her feet gently with your own warm hands.

27. You are called to the home of a 16-year-old boy who has attempted suicide by inhaling carbon monoxide. Upon arrival, you find the garage door open, the boy unconscious and slumped over the steering wheel of a running automobile, and the parents shaking the boy. You see that the boy is still breathing. Your first step in this situation would be to remove the boy from the garage and then:

    A. begin CPR.

    B. give 100% oxygen.

    C. give a 50% oxygen mixture to the boy.

    D. place the boy in a side-lying position.

28. The diving reflex can occur when:

    A. a person dives into shallow water.

    B. a person jumps or dives into very cold water.

    C. the extremities lose feeling in very cold water.

    D. the body is immersed in water deeper than 6 feet.

29. An electric shock can cause cardiac arrest because the shock may cause:

    A. the blood vessels to dilate.

    B. the blood vessels to constrict.

    C. the heart muscle to contract.

    D. a disruption of the heart's normal electrical rhythm.

Environmental Injuries

30. Your care for a patient who has received an electric shock should begin with making certain that the power has been turned off, followed by:

    A. moving the patient to a flat surface.

    B. giving a painful stimulus.

    C. checking for respirations and pulse.

    D. assessing for injuries.

31. Treatment of a chemical burn to the eye should include:

    A. covering both the injured and uninjured eyes and providing transport.

    B. irrigating the injured eye with a commercial eyewash preparation.

    C. irrigating the injured eye with water for 5 to 20 minutes.

    D. neutralizing the chemical, then flushing the eye with water.

32. Alkali burns are more serious than acid burns because alkali:

    A. lacerates the skin, causing heavy bleeding.

    B. penetrates more deeply into the tissues.

    C. cannot be washed off easily.

    D. causes flash burns.

33. A 10-year-old boy who was playing with matches set his clothes on fire. His skin is blistering and leathery, and you see several charred areas on his skin. The patient's burns should be classified as:

    A. first-degree burns.

    B. first- and second-degree burns.

    C. second- and third-degree burns.

    D. third-degree burns.

Chapter 20

34. A third-degree burn is also called:

    A. a partial-thickness burn.

    B. a full-thickness burn.

    C. a semi-thickness burn.

    D. an ultra-thickness burn.

35. The purpose of the Rule of Nines is to:

    A. estimate the amount of body surface area affected.

    B. estimate the degree of burn.

    C. describe the patient's condition.

    D. describe the section of the body involved.

36. The subcutaneous layer of the skin functions as:

    A. a waterproof layer.

    B. a barrier against bacteria.

    C. an insulator for the body.

    D. storage for pigment cells.

37. Sweat and oil glands are located in the:

    A. dermis.

    B. epidermis.

    C. muscle fascia.

    D. muscle layer.

38. Artificial ventilation for a patient involved in a near-drowning accident should begin as soon as the patient is:

    A. moved into the ambulance.

    B. pulled from the water and placed on a firm surface.

    C. pulled from the water and placed on a spine board.

    D. positioned faceup in the water.

Environmental Injuries

39. The first step in treating a burn patient is to:

    A. provide immediate transport.

    B. stop further burning from occurring.

    C. apply moist, sterile dressings.

    D. apply dry, sterile dressings.

40. In patients with severe burns, shock usually results from:

    A. fluid loss.

    B. emotional distress.

    C. anxiety.

    D. pain.

41. Emergency treatment of thermal burns of the eyelids should include:

    A. irrigating the eyes with water for 15 minutes.

    B. irrigating the eyes with a commercial preparation.

    C. covering the eyes with moist sterile, dressings.

    D. covering the eyes with dry, sterile dressings.

42. Key factors that determine the seriousness of thermal burns include:

    A. determination of burn thickness and amount of blood loss.

    B. depth of the burn and amount of body surface area involved.

    C. height and weight of the patient.

    D. the patient's age and amount of blood loss.

Chapter 20

43. When a patient's skin has been burned by an unknown liquid acid or alkali, you should:

    A. provide immediate transport with the patient in a side-lying position.

    B. neutralize the substance with a mild solution of the opposite pH, then flush the skin with water for 20 minutes.

    C. irrigate the skin with water for 20 minutes, then neutralize the substance with a mild solution of the opposite pH.

    D. irrigate the skin with copious amounts of water until the burning has stopped, and then continue irrigating for an additional 10 minutes.

44. An inhaled poison will enter the body through the:

    A. body tissues.

    B. digestive tract.

    C. respiratory tract.

    D. bloodstream.

45. Treatment of an animal or human bite should include:

    A. applying a dry, sterile dressing and providing prompt transport to the emergency department.

    B. applying a constricting band above and below the wound.

    C. washing the wound with Mercurochrome or Merthiolate.

    D. washing the wound with alcohol.

46. An area of burned skin that is still burning can be made less painful by:

    A. immersing the area in cool water.

    B. covering the area with a sterile burn pad.

    C. covering the area with a waterless type of ointment.

    D. spraying the area with a burn ointment.

Environmental Injuries

47. Characteristics of first-degree burns include:

    A. red skin and pain.

    B. red skin and blisters.

    C. blisters and no pain.

    D. charred, dry, leathery skin.

48. A person submerged in water colder than 70°F may develop:

    A. hypoxia.

    B. laryngospasm.

    C. hyperthermia.

    D. hypothermia.

49. When a person is submerged in cold water, the temperature of the water will cause the patient's:

    A. heart rate to increase and respirations to become shallow.

    B. heart rate to increase and respirations to deepen.

    C. metabolism to slow down and the need for oxygen to decrease.

    D. blood to be concentrated in the extremities.

50. Carbon monoxide is a poison that is:

    A. inhaled.

    B. ingested.

    C. injected.

    D. absorbed.

Chapter 20

Answers

1: **D.** Carbon monoxide is a colorless, odorless gas that combines with hemoglobin in the blood, blocking the transport of oxygen to body tissues. (ECTSI 5, p. 35)

2: **D.** Management of hypothermia in the field focuses on stabilizing the vital signs and preventing further heat loss. (ECTSI 5, p. 630)

3: **C.** Gamma rays are considered the most dangerous type of ionizing radiation. (ECTSI 5, p. 609)

4: **B.** The greatest danger of beta rays is the accidental contact or ingestion of beta-radioactive materials. (ECTSI 5, p. 609)

5: **C.** When called to treat a patient injured in an accident in which he or she is exposed to radiation and the source of radiation is still present, you should first put on protective clothing and then rapidly move the patient out of danger. (ECTSI 5, p. 611)

6: **A.** Move a burn patient away from the burning area to prevent any further injury. If the patient's skin is still burning, immerse the burned skin in cool water for no more than 10 minutes. (ECTSI 5, p. 601)

7: **D.** The Rule of Nines is modified for an infant, because an infant's head takes up relatively more body surface area than an adult's, and the legs take up less. (ECTSI 5, p. 600)

8: **B.** The greatest danger to a patient who has sustained a burn is the possibility of infection. (ECTSI 5, p. 601)

9: **C.** Shivering in the presence of hypothermia indicates that the body is trying to generate more heat through muscular activity. (ECTSI 5, p. 629)

10: **A.** Emergency treatment of heatstroke concentrates on decreasing the patient's body temperature. (ECTSI 5, p. 628)

11: **D.** A patient with hypothermia has lost the ability to regulate body temperature and generate body heat. (ECTSI 5, p. 629)

12: **B.** The best way to ease the pain of light burns to the eye is to cover each eye with sterile, moist pads and an eye shield. Transport the patient to the hospital in a supine position. (ECTSI 5, p. 358)

Environmental Injuries

13: **A.** Emergency treatment for both air embolism and decompression sickness is providing basic life support measures and providing transport to the nearest recompression chamber. (ECTSI 5, p. 641)

14: **A.** Rotate the upper half of the body as a unit until the patient is faceup. Clear the airway and then begin rescue breathing. (ECTSI 5, p. 638)

15: **B.** One result of severe hypothermia is the possibility of cardiac arrhythmia. (ECTSI 5, p. 630)

16: **D.** The amount of radiation exposure that a person receives depends on the distance of the person from the radiation source. (ECTSI 5, p. 609)

17: **B.** Even if initial field resuscitation of a near-drowning patient appears to be completely successful, the patient should be transported to the emergency department to check for fluid aspiration. (ECTSI 5, p. 637)

18: **A.** Treatment of a patient with heat exhaustion should include moving him to a cool area, treating him for hypovolemic shock, and encouraging him to drink up to a liter of water. (ECTSI 5, p. 627)

19: **B.** You should suspect heatstroke when the patient's skin is hot and dry, and his temperature is elevated. (ECTSI 5, p. 627)

20: **D.** The principal goal in treatment of heat exposure is to reduce the patient's body temperature. (ECTSI 5, pp. 626–627)

21: **C.** If it is necessary to rewarm a frostbitten extremity in the field (In this situation, the patient has been moved to a warm environment.), it should be done by immersing the affected part in water at a temperature of between 100° and 112°F. (ECTSI 5, p. 632)

22: **B.** Never give up on resuscitating a drowning victim. Submersion in very cold water will produce hypothermia, which protects the vital organs from lack of oxygen. Once the child has been removed from the water, you should clear the airway and then begin CPR. (ECTSI 5, p. 639)

23: **B.** A general definition of hypothermia is progressive cooling of the body. (ECTSI 5, p. 629)

24: **C.** Treatment of hypothermia at the scene includes removing the patient from the cold environment to prevent further heat loss. (ECTSI 5, p. 630)

25: **D.** Frostnip occurs when the skin freezes but deeper tissues do not. (ECTSI 5, p. 631)

Chapter 20

26: **A.** When treating a patient with frostbite, you should remove any wet clothing and cover the affected part or parts with a dry, sterile dressing. (ECTSI 5, p. 632)

27: **B.** The first step in caring for this patient is to move him from the area and then administer 100% oxygen. (ECTSI 5, p. 602)

28: **B.** The diving reflex can occur when a person jumps or dives into very cold water. (ECTSI 5, p. 639)

29: **D.** The energy from an electric shock may disrupt the heart's normal rhythm and cause cardiac arrest. (ECTSI 5, p. 605)

30: **C.** After making certain that the power source has been turned off, the next step in treating a patient who has received an electric shock is to check for respirations and pulse, followed by CPR, if necessary. (ECTSI 5, p. 607)

31: **C.** Irrigate the eye with water for at least 5 minutes if it has been splashed with an acid chemical, and for 10 to 20 minutes if it has been splashed with an alkali chemical. (ECTSI 5, p. 604)

32: **B.** Alkali burns are more serious than acid burns because alkalis will penetrate more deeply into tissues. (ECTSI 5, p. 603)

33: **C.** A patient with blistering and leathery, charred areas of skin has second- and third-degree burns. Second-degree burns are characterized by blister formation. Third-degree burns are characterized by dry, leathery, and charred or chalk-white skin. (ECTSI 5, p. 599)

34: **B.** A third-degree burn is also called a full-thickness burn. (ECTSI 5, p. 600)

35: **A.** The Rule of Nines is used to estimate the amount of body surface damage sustained in a burn. (ECTSI 5, p. 600)

36: **C.** The subcutaneous layer of the skin is composed largely of fat, which acts as an insulator for the body. (ECTSI 5, p. 597)

37: **A.** Sweat and oil glands are located in the dermis, along with hair follicles, blood vessels, and specialized nerve endings. (ECTSI 5, p. 597)

38: **D.** Artificial ventilation for a patient involved in a near-drowning accident should begin as soon as possible, even while the patient is still in the water. (ECTSI 5, p. 636)

Environmental Injuries

39: **B.** The first step in treating a burn patient is to stop any further burning from occurring. (ECTSI 5, p. 601)

40: **A.** Shock usually results from fluid loss in patients with severe burns. (ECTSI 5, p. 210)

41: **C.** Emergency treatment of thermal burns to the eyelids should include covering the eyes with moist, sterile dressings and transporting the patient. (ECTSI 5, p. 357)

42: **B.** Key factors that determine the seriousness of thermal burns include the depth of the burn and the amount of surface area involved. Also included are the involvement of critical areas and the patient's age and general health. (ECTSI 5, p. 600)

43: **D.** Treatment of a patient who has been burned by an unknown liquid acid or alkali should include flushing the area with water until the burning stops, and then continuing flushing for another 10 minutes. (ECTSI 5, p. 603)

44: **C.** An inhaled poison enters the body through the respiratory tract. (ECTSI 5, p. 602)

45: **A.** Treatment of an animal or human bite in the field consists of the application of a dry, sterile dressing and prompt transport to the emergency department. In addition, for a human bite, the injured area should be immobilized. (ECTSI 5, pp. 442–443)

46: **A.** A burned area of skin that is still burning can be made less painful by immersing it in cool water, or by covering it with a cool, wet dressing. (ECTSI 5, p. 601)

47: **A.** First-degree burns are characterized by red skin and pain. (ECTSI 5, p. 599)

48: **D.** Hypothermia may occur if a person is submerged in water colder than 70°F. (ECTSI 5, p. 639)

49: **C.** Metabolism will slow down and the need for oxygen will decrease if a person is submerged in cold water. (ECTSI 5, p. 639)

50: **A.** Carbon monoxide is a poison that is inhaled. (ECTSI 5, p. 602)

Chapter 21

Poisons, Stings, and Bites

Chapter Goals

The exercises in this chapter are designed to help the student to:

- identify the different routes of poisoning.

- identify the signs and symptoms of poisoning and the most likely toxic substance.

- describe appropriate emergency care for different types of poisoning, including swallowed, inhaled, injected, and surface poisons, food poisoning, and plant poisoning.

- identify the signs and symptoms of stings from insects and spiders.

- identify the signs and symptoms of anaphylaxis.

- describe appropriate emergency care for anaphylaxis.

Poisons, Stings, and Bites

Multiple-Choice Questions

Select the correct answer for each of the following questions. Each question has only *one* correct or best answer.

1. Your immediate treatment of a man who is disoriented, stuporous, and drifting in and out of consciousness as a result of swallowing 30 sleeping pills should consist of:

    A. diluting the poison while waiting for instructions from poison control.

    B. covering the patient with a blanket and then placing him in a side-lying position while waiting for him to vomit.

    C. providing immediate transport and giving supplemental oxygen en route to the hospital.

    D. inducing vomiting while waiting for further instructions from medical control.

2. A woman states that she has taken an "overdose of a downer." Your care of this patient should begin with:

    A. trying to "talk her down."

    B. trying to prevent her from injuring herself.

    C. maintaining an airway and providing respiratory support.

    D. referring her to her personal physician for a dependency problem.

3. In which of the following situations is it impossible to remove or dilute the poisoning substance?

    A. A teenager has swallowed 20 sleeping pills.

    B. A factory worker has backed into a bag of dry fertilizer.

    C. A man has been overcome by ammonia fumes.

    D. A woman has been bitten by a black widow spider.

Chapter 21

4. Constricting bands placed above and below the site of a snakebite injury should stop the flow of:

    A. capillary blood.

    B. both arterial and venous blood.

    C. arterial blood, but not venous blood.

    D. venous blood, but not arterial blood.

5. Which of the following assessment findings commonly appears in patients who have had an anaphylactic reaction?

    A. Hives

    B. Chills

    C. Severe nausea

    D. Hypertension

6. Which of the following assessment findings indicate that a patient may be going into anaphylactic shock?

    A. Slow, strong pulse, dizziness, cold sweats, nausea

    B. Weak pulse, itchy, red skin, shallow breathing

    C. Blank expression, cold extremities, normal breathing

    D. Blank expression, chills, unconsciousness, dry skin

7. A teenage girl states that she was stung on the arm and that she knows she is allergic to bee stings. You see a wheal on the arm at the site of the sting. To slow the spread of the toxin, you should place which of the following directly over the site?

    A. An ice bag

    B. A warm compress

    C. A constricting band

    D. A saline-moistened dressing

236 Student Review Manual

Poisons, Stings, and Bites

8. A patient is alert and conscious after ingesting an unknown quantity of "some pills." The first step in caring for this patient should be to:

   A. call medical control for instructions.

   B. treat the patient for shock and then call poison control.

   C. induce vomiting and then call poison control.

   D. provide immediate transport to the emergency department.

9. A 19-year-old man who is bitten on the leg by a rattlesnake is found sitting on the ground leaning against a tree. The patient is weak and sweaty and states that his leg is burning. As you begin your assessment the patient vomits and becomes very anxious. Your care for this patient should begin by:

   A. giving him small sips of water to clear his mouth.

   B. placing a venous constricting band directly over the bite area.

   C. placing venous constricting bands above and below the bite area.

   D. placing a warm compress over the bite area.

10. You are called to the home of a 3-year-old child who has had severe abdominal pain, nausea, and vomiting for the past 24 hours. The child has also been feverish and weak. The parents state that the child's grandmother and cousin have had the same symptoms since a family picnic 2 days ago. The most appropriate course of action would be to:

    A. tell the parents to give the child plenty of water to drink and call their personal physician if the child does not improve in 24 hours.

    B. tell the parents that the child has botulism food poisoning and that the poison will have to "run its course."

    C. perform a thorough assessment and provide transport to the hospital.

    D. give the child plenty of water to drink and then call poison control.

Chapter 21

11. An 18-year-old man has ingested a bottle of an alkali drain cleaner in a suicide attempt. The patient is conscious and complaining that his mouth is burning. The first step in caring for this patient would be to give him:

    A. vinegar to drink to neutralize the alkali.

    B. syrup of ipecac and monitor his airway.

    C. milk, then syrup of ipecac, and call poison control.

    D. water and call poison control.

12. A 52-year-old woman who has a heart condition has taken an accidental overdose of her medication. Upon your arrival, she is conscious and alert. Of the following, the best course of action is to give her:

    A. water and call poison control.

    B. water and induce vomiting.

    C. syrup of ipecac immediately.

    D. oxygen and then provide transport.

13. A hiker has an extremely swollen, painful leg after being bitten by a rattlesnake. Field management of this patient should include applying:

    A. venous constricting bands above and below the site, at the edge of the swelling.

    B. a venous constricting band above the site of the swelling.

    C. a venous constricting band below the site of the swelling.

    D. tourniquets above and below the site of the swelling.

Poisons, Stings, and Bites

14. You are called to the home of an elderly woman who states that she is having difficulty breathing and her chest feels "tight." The back of her left leg has been numb for several hours, and she has had severe abdominal cramps. During your assessment, the woman says that she was fine until after she started cleaning in the garage yesterday, but claims that she did not do any heavy lifting. The back of her leg looks normal except for a light pink rash and what appear to be two small puncture wounds. Your care of the patient should include:

    A. placing warm compresses on the leg, giving oxygen, and then providing transport.

    B. placing ice on the leg and advising the patient to call her physician.

    C. applying venous constricting bands above and below the site of the rash, giving oxygen, and then providing transport.

    D. giving oxygen, and then transporting the patient for further examination.

15. You are called to a playground where a 5-year-old boy has been bitten by a dog. The child is crying and holding his bleeding arm. Other children at the playground tell you, "Eric's dog bit Steve." You also learn that the child's mother is on her way to the playground. Treatment at the scene should begin with:

    A. washing the wound with an antiseptic soap and covering it with a cold compress.

    B. washing the wound with an antiseptic soap and placing an ice pack on the area to prevent swelling.

    C. splinting the arm and covering the wound with a moistened sterile dressing.

    D. covering the wound with a dry, sterile dressing and providing transport.

16. Carbon monoxide produces death by:

    A. overstimulating the central nervous system.

    B. destroying the alveoli in the lungs.

    C. combining with hemoglobin and reducing the amount of oxygen reaching the cells.

    D. combining with white blood cells and preventing oxygen from reaching the cells.

Chapter 21

17. An 18-month-old boy is found sitting on the kitchen floor with an empty bottle of furniture polish and a half-empty bottle of lighter fluid lying next to him. The child is conscious and alert. Your first step in caring for this patient should be to:

    A. give him a "double" dose of syrup of ipecac to induce vomiting.

    B. give the patient plenty of water to drink and then call poison control for instructions.

    C. try to absorb the poison by giving the patient activated charcoal mixed into a bottle of water.

    D. ask the parent why the patient had access to these poisons as you try to induce vomiting.

18. A 5-year-old girl was stung several times by a swarm of bees. The areas where she was stung are red and swollen, and several stingers are embedded in the arms, legs, and face. The patient is crying and complains of severe pain in the area surrounding each sting. The parents state that she has no known allergy to bee stings. The patient has a rapid pulse. The most appropriate course of action would be to:

    A. try to pull out all of the stingers, apply warm compresses to the areas, then provide transport.

    B. try to pull out all of the stingers, apply ice packs to the areas, then provide transport.

    C. apply warm compresses to the areas, give oxygen, then provide transport.

    D. apply ice packs to the areas, then provide immediate transport.

19. Syrup of ipecac should be used in treating a poisoning victim in which of the following situations?

    A. All cases of suspected poisoning by ingestion

    B. When it is necessary to induce vomiting

    C. When the patient has swallowed an acid

    D. When no other means of treatment is available

Poisons, Stings, and Bites

20. A child has swallowed an unknown number of leaves from a green house plant. Upon your arrival, she is conscious and alert. The best course of action would be to:

    A. give her syrup of ipecac immediately.

    B. treat her for shock and provide immediate transport.

    C. give her plenty of water to drink, call poison control and ask if you should induce vomiting.

    D. give her plenty of water to drink and advise the parents to call their personal physician if the child becomes ill.

21. A 13-year-old boy has muscle cramps and burning pain in his left arm after spending the night sleeping in a tent in his backyard. There are two red dots just below the elbow, and discoloration and swelling in the area around the elbow. The patient is sweating and has tightness across the chest and some difficulty breathing. He has a blood pressure of 100/70 mm Hg, a pulse of 100/min, and labored respirations of 18/min. The patient's signs and symptoms suggest that he was bitten by a:

    A. rattlesnake.

    B. coral snake.

    C. black widow spider.

    D. brown recluse spider.

22. A man is found unconscious in his car with the window open. His face is severely swollen and he is barely breathing. A law enforcement officer at the scene tells you that he saw the man's car slow down and then park at the side of the road. You should first:

    A. search for an epinephrine kit in the car.

    B. give oxygen and prepare to perform CPR, if necessary.

    C. place cool compresses on the face and provide immediate transport.

    D. look for an embedded stinger and then pull it out before providing transport.

Chapter 21

23. A 14-year-old boy has severe burning pain on the back of his right wrist that extends to his elbow after being bitten by an unidentified snake. The area around the fang marks is swollen, as is the rest of the arm up to the elbow. The patient has a blood pressure of 100/70 mm Hg, a pulse of 110/min, and respirations of 20/min. As you prepare to transport the patient, you should first:

    A. give him oxygen and place him in a supine position.

    B. cover the wound with a dry, sterile dressing and then splint the extremity.

    C. place venous constricting bands above and below the fang marks.

    D. place venous constricting bands above and below the fang marks, cover the wound with a warm compress, and give oxygen.

24. Which of the following infectious diseases is spread as a result of a tick bite?

    A. Rabies

    B. Malaria

    C. Hepatitis B

    D. Lyme disease

25. Symptoms of food poisoning caused by which of the following organisms usually develop within 1 to 3 hours after the food was consumed?

    A. Clostridium

    B. Staphylococcus

    C. Salmonella

    D. Streptococcus

Poisons, Stings, and Bites

Answers

1: **C.** A patient who is drifting in and out of consciousness after barbiturate poisoning should be considered a real emergency. Therefore, immediate treatment should consist of providing immediate transport and giving supplemental oxygen en route to the hospital. Inducing vomiting in a patient who is semiconscious or unconscious is very dangerous, as it may result in aspiration. (ECTSI 5, p. 428)

2: **C.** "Downers" depress the central nervous system. Therefore, care of this patient should begin with ensuring that the airway remains clear and providing respiratory support if necessary. (ECTSI 5, p. 428)

3: **D.** Of the situations listed, only the black widow spider bite cannot be removed or diluted. An injected poison is essentially impossible to remove from the bloodstream, although placing venous constricting bands or applying ice to the area can slow the absorption of the toxin. In each of the other situations, it is possible to remove or dilute the poison. (ECTSI 5, p. 429)

4: **D.** Constricting bands placed above and below the site of a snakebite injury should stop the flow of venous blood, but not arterial blood. (ECTSI 5, p. 439)

5: **A.** One of the most common signs of an anaphylactic reaction is urticaria or hives. (ECTSI 5, p. 433)

6: **B.** Weak pulse, itchy, red skin, and shallow breathing are all signs that a patient may be going into anaphylactic shock. (ECTSI 5, pp. 211, 433)

7: **A.** To slow the spread of the toxin from a bee sting, you should place an ice pack over the site of the sting. (ECTSI 5, p. 434)

8: **A.** If the patient is conscious, you should first call medical control for instructions. Dispatch will generally contact the poison control center and relay instructions. (ECTSI 5, p. 426)

9: **C.** The first steps in caring for a patient who has been bitten by a pit viper such as a rattlesnake are to place venous constricting bands above and below the bite area as you reassure the patient that poisonous snakebites rarely cause death. (ECTSI 5, p. 439)

Chapter 21

10: **C.** With instances of possible food poisoning, you should perform a thorough assessment and then provide transport to the emergency department where the patient can be examined by a physician. In suspected botulism, you may have to assist respirations and give basic life support, if necessary. (ECTSI 5, p. 430)

11: **D.** The first step in caring for a conscious patient who has ingested an alkali is to dilute the poison with milk or water and then call poison control for further instructions. (ECTSI 5, pp. 427–428)

12: **A.** The best course of action when a patient who takes an accidental overdose of a nonbarbiturate, but is still conscious and alert, is to dilute the poison and then call poison control for further instructions. (ECTSI 5, pp. 427–428)

13: **A.** Field management of a patient with a rattlesnake bite to an extremity should include applying venous constricting bands above and below the site of the fang marks, at the edge of the swelling. (ECTSI 5, p. 439)

14: **D.** These findings suggest a black widow spider bite, and because the patient is experiencing respiratory problems, she should be given oxygen and taken to the hospital. Applying constricting bands would not be appropriate for this patient. (ECTSI 5, p. 435)

15: **D.** Prehospital care for dog bites consists of placing a dry, sterile dressing over the wound and then providing transport to the emergency department. Because rabies is always a concern, the dog should be located as soon as possible by law enforcement or animal control officers for evaluation. (ECTSI 5, p. 442)

16: **C.** Carbon monoxide produces death by combining with hemoglobin and reducing the amount of oxygen reaching the cells. (ECTSI 5, p. 35)

17: **B.** The first step in caring for a patient who has swallowed a petroleum product, such as furniture polish and/or lighter fluid is to dilute the poison and call poison control. You should not attempt to induce vomiting because these agents will cause a serious chemical pneumonia if their vapors are inhaled or aspirated. (ECTSI 5, p. 428)

18: **D.** The most appropriate course of action in this situation would be to apply ice to the sting areas and provide immediate transport. You should not attempt to remove stingers in this situation where, even though the patient is not known to be allergic, she has received a massive dose of bee venom. Application of ice may help to relieve some of the pain. (ECTSI 5, p. 432)

Poisons, Stings, and Bites

19: **B.** Syrup of ipecac is used when it is necessary to induce vomiting. (ECTSI 5, p. 428)

20: **C.** The best course of action for a suspected plant poisoning is to dilute the poison, then call poison control to ask if you should induce vomiting. (ECTSI 5, pp. 430–431)

21: **C.** This patient's signs and symptoms suggest that he was bitten by a black widow spider. (ECTSI 5, p. 435)

22: **B.** The first steps in caring for a patient who has apparently had a severe anaphylactic reaction are to give oxygen and prepare to perform CPR if he stops breathing and has no pulse. Basic life support measures and immediate transport to the emergency department are most important in this situation. (ECTSI 5, p. 434)

23: **C.** The patient shows signs and symptoms that envenomation has occurred. He has severe burning pain and swelling. As you prepare to transport the patient, you should place venous constricting bands above and below the fang marks to slow the absorption of the toxin. (ECTSI 5, p. 439)

24: **D.** Lyme disease is spread by ticks, as is Rocky Mountain spotted fever. Lyme disease is caused by an infecting bacterium that is carried by a tick, not by the bite itself. (ECTSI 5, p. 441)

25: **B.** Symptoms of food poisoning caused by *Staphylococcus* bacterium usually develop within 1 to 3 hours after the food was consumed. (ECTSI 5, p. 430)

Chapter 22

Interacting With Patients

Chapter Goals

The exercises in this chapter are designed to help the student to:

- explain the principles of effective communication.

- list specific communication problems and how to solve them.

- describe how to manage a disruptive patient.

Interacting With Patients

Multiple-Choice Questions

Select the correct answer for each of the following questions. Each question has only *one* correct or best answer.

1. A patient who believes that others (including you) are plotting to hurt or kill him is most likely:

    A. manic.

    B. suicidal.

    C. paranoid.

    D. depressed.

2. A patient who is alert, oriented, and thinking clearly should be described as:

    A. lucid.

    B. manic.

    C. normal.

    D. conscious.

3. The best way to communicate with a frightened patient is to:

    A. shout at her.

    B. use medical terminology.

    C. assure her that she will be fine.

    D. make and keep eye contact with her.

4. A patient who refuses to cooperate and will not answer your questions is most likely experiencing:

    A. a psychotic episode.

    B. depression.

    C. euphoria.

    D. mania.

Chapter 22

5. An important step to take in the management of a disruptive patient is to:

    A. provide proper emergency medical care as soon as it is safe to do so.

    B. lecture the patient about causing a delay in treatment.

    C. allow the patient to take charge of the situation.

    D. tell the patient you do not care for drunks.

6. The driver in a one-car accident has no apparent injuries, but she is acting unruly. A half-full whiskey bottle is lying on the passenger seat. The appropriate course of action would be to:

    A. assume that the driver is drunk.

    B. let law enforcement officials handle the matter.

    C. ask bystanders to help you restrain the driver.

    D. assess the situation to determine why the driver is acting unruly.

7. A patient with organic brain syndrome who is exhibiting disruptive behavior will most likely be:

    A. unable to speak.

    B. terminally ill.

    C. elderly.

    D. paralyzed.

8. A woman is extremely agitated and moving around frantically. She is speaking rapidly, but does not finish her sentences. These signs and symptoms suggest:

    A. mania.

    B. paranoia.

    C. depression.

    D. a potential suicide attempt.

Interacting With Patients

9. The first step in the management of a patient exhibiting disruptive behavior is to:

    A. call the police.

    B. assess the situation.

    C. give supplemental oxygen.

    D. notify the emergency department.

10. A patient who is malingering is generally considered to be:

    A. in the last stages of a terminal illness.

    B. not getting enough vitamins.

    C. having gastric reflux.

    D. faking illness.

11. Your primary responsibility in the initial management of a disruptive patient is to:

    A. make a specific diagnosis.

    B. take charge of the situation, but protect yourself if necessary.

    C. lecture the patient about the dangers of substance abuse.

    D. protect yourself so if the patient harms himself it is his own fault.

12. If a patient does not speak English, you should:

    A. seek out a family member or friend to interpret.

    B. speak slowly so the patient can understand you.

    C. transfer the patient without speaking to him.

    D. call the police for back-up.

13. "Patronizing" a patient means that you:

    A. lie to the patient.

    B. use sign language to ask questions.

    C. touch the patient in an inappropriate manner.

    D. use language and behavior that is not respectful to the patient.

Chapter 22

14. As you begin caring for an injured child, remember that the child:

    A. should be kept away from the parents.

    B. will be frightened.

    C. need not be told what you are doing.

    D. need not be told that treatment might hurt.

15. If you have been directed by the police to restrain a disruptive patient, you should:

    A. use police handcuffs.

    B. use whatever means are available.

    C. use soft, wide leather or cloth restraints.

    D. refuse to do it and let the police handle it.

16. For some people, disruptive behavior is a natural response:

    A. especially among women.

    B. especially among men.

    C. to authority figures.

    D. to stress.

17. Treatment of a patient who is mentally retarded should be handled:

    A. by a mental health professional only.

    B. by at least three EMTs because the patient may become disruptive.

    C. in a way that will minimize the patient's fear and confusion.

    D. in a way that will make communicating with the patient unnecessary.

Interacting With Patients

18. Make sure you are careful of what you say to others in the presence of an unresponsive patient because:

    A. information about the patient is confidential.

    B. the patient's family need not know the nature of the patient's condition.

    C. the patient may hear only part of the conversation and misinterpret your statements.

    D. the patient is your only concern and you should direct all of your comments to the patient.

19. The proper way to speak with a patient who is hearing impaired is to:

    A. shout so the patient can hear you.

    B. use sign language only so the patient will not be embarrassed.

    C. position yourself so the patient can read your lips and then speak clearly and slowly.

    D. communicate through family members because the patient may be mentally retarded.

20. The proper way to assess an elderly patient is to:

    A. use a calm, slow approach and allow plenty of time for the patient to respond to your questions.

    B. use more compassion than with other patients because the patient is likely to be in pain.

    C. focus only on clinical signs to avoid being misled by inaccurate information from family members.

    D. make decisions independently of what the patient may say, because the patient is probably not thinking rationally.

Chapter 22

21. Which of the following represents the proper way to lead a patient who is blind but is able to walk to the ambulance?

    A. Stay in physical contact with the patient, placing your hand on the patient's shoulder or arm and explain what is happening.

    B. Guide the patient by gently pushing on the patient's back and explain what is happening.

    C. Guide the patient by gently pushing on the patient, assuming that the patient is also hearing impaired and/or mentally retarded.

    D. Ask the patient to leave his or her seeing-eye dog at home and then guide the patient yourself.

22. In sign language, both hands closed with the index fingers extended pointing toward one another in front of your chest means:

    A. sick.

    B. hurt.

    C. help.

    D. call 911.

Answers

1: **C.** A patient who is paranoid may believe that you or others are plotting to hurt or kill him. (ECTSI 5, p. 652)

2: **A.** A patient who is alert, oriented, and thinking clearly should be described as lucid. (ECTSI 5, p. 652)

3: **D.** The best way to communicate with a frightened patient is to make and keep eye contact in order to help the patient keep calm. (ECTSI 5, p. 647)

4: **B.** A patient who is experiencing depression may not want to do anything, be cooperative, or answer questions. (ECTSI 5, p. 652)

5: **A.** Providing proper emergency medical care as soon as it is safe to do so is an important step in the management of a disruptive patient. (ECTSI 5, p. 652)

6: **D.** The appropriate course of action in this situation would be to assess the scene to determine why the driver is being disruptive. It is not your job to make assumptions about legal intoxication. (ECTSI 5, pp. 651–653)

Interacting With Patients

7: **C.** Most patients with organic brain syndrome are elderly. (ECTSI 5, p. 651)

8: **A.** Extreme agitation, quick disjointed movement, and the inability to finish thoughts are classic signs of a manic state. (ECTSI 5, p. 652)

9: **B.** The first step in the management of a patient exhibiting disruptive behavior is to assess the situation. (ECTSI 5, p. 652)

10: **D.** A patient who is malingering is generally considered to be faking illness. (ECTSI 5, p. 653)

11: **B.** Your primary responsibility in the initial management of a disruptive patient is to take charge of the situation and to be mindful of your personal safety. (ECTSI 5, p. 652)

12: **A.** You should seek out a family member or friend to interpret when a patient does not speak English. (ECTSI 5, p. 650)

13: **D.** You should communicate with a patient at a level the patient can understand without talking down to or "patronizing" the patient or telling a lie. (ECTSI 5, p. 647)

14: **B.** You should assume that an injured child will be frightened. (ECTSI 5, pp. 648–649)

15: **C.** Whenever the police ask you to restrain a patient, you should use only soft, wide leather or cloth restraints, not police handcuffs. (ECTSI 5, p. 653)

16: **D.** Although there are many causes of disruptive behavior, for some people it is simply a natural reaction to stress. Disruptive behavior is not a "natural" gender-specific reaction. (ECTSI 5, p. 651)

17: **C.** Treatment of a patient who is mentally retarded should be handled with caring concern in order to minimize fear and confusion. (ECTSI 5, p. 651)

18: **C.** An unresponsive patient may hear part or all of what you say and seriously misinterpret your statements. (ECTSI 5, p. 648)

19: **C.** Whenever you are assessing the condition of a patient with a hearing impairment, position yourself so the patient can see your lips, and then make sure you speak clearly and slowly. (ECTSI 5, p. 649)

20: **A.** Whenever you are assessing an elderly patient's condition, use a calm, slow approach and allow plenty of time for response to your questions. (ECTSI 5, p. 648)

Chapter 22

21: **A.** The proper way to guide a person who is blind is to place your hand on the person's shoulder or arm, maintaining physical contact but not pushing. Also stay in constant communication with the person. (ECTSI 5, p. 649)

22: **B.** This gesture means "hurt." It is helpful for the EMT to know some of the simple phrases used in sign language, including those for "sick," "hurt," and "help." (ECTSI 5, pp. 649–650)

Chapter 23

Crisis Intervention

Chapter Goals

The exercises in this chapter are designed to help the student to:

- describe techniques for dealing with sudden death.

- describe how to care for a patient who is terminally ill.

- explain how to care for a patient who has been abused or assaulted.

- list the signs of child abuse and how to treat them.

- identify the various legal documents regarding a patient's dying wishes.

- identify signs of sudden infant death syndrome (SIDS) and how to care for the family.

- describe Critical Incident Stress Debriefing (CISD) and how it works.

Chapter 23

Multiple-Choice Questions

Select the correct answer for each of the following questions. Each question has only *one* correct or best answer.

1. Of the following, which individual can legally pronounce a patient dead?

    A. A police officer

    B. A registered nurse

    C. A licensed physician

    D. An emergency medical technician

2. Which of the following conclusive signs of death occurs when dependent body parts turn bluish-red or purple due to blood settling to the lower parts of the body?

    A. Lividity

    B. Rigor mortis

    C. Decapitation

    D. Decomposition

3. Which of the following conclusive signs of death occurs when the entire body stiffens several hours after death?

    A. Lividity

    B. Rigor mortis

    C. Decapitation

    D. Decomposition

4. What are the four phases of emotional response commonly experienced by patients who have a terminal illness?

    A. Denial, anger, paranoia, and grief

    B. Denial, anger, paranoia, and acceptance

    C. Denial, anger, depression, and grief

    D. Denial, anger, depression, and acceptance

Crisis Intervention

5. The laws in most states recognize that a statement or statements made by a patient who knows he or she is dying are accepted as legal documents or sworn statements. This type of statement is commonly called a:

    A. confession.

    B. living will.

    C. sworn statement.

    D. dying declaration.

6. When treating a patient who has been raped, you should:

    A. avoid examining the patient's genitalia for any reason.

    B. avoid examining the patient's genitalia unless there is obvious bleeding.

    C. make sure to examine the patient's genitalia for injury and evidence.

    D. make sure to ask the patient for permission to examine the genitalia for evidence.

7. How can you distinguish between a gesture for help by a patient and a serious suicide attempt?

    A. You will not be able to distinguish the difference.

    B. You will be able to tell by the seriousness of the injury.

    C. You must rely on communication from the patient.

    D. You must rely on communication from the patient's family.

8. The first step in the treatment of suspected child abuse is to:

    A. call law enforcement officials to the scene.

    B. encourage the alleged abuser to seek counseling.

    C. remove the child from the environment producing the abuse.

    D. preserve the chain of evidence needed to help convict the alleged abuser.

Chapter 23

9. Sudden infant death syndrome (SIDS) usually occurs in children between the ages of:

    A. 10 to 30 days.

    B. 2 to 4 months.

    C. 6 to 8 months.

    D. 10 to 18 months.

10. You have been called to the scene of an automobile accident. The passenger in the front seat was not wearing his seat belt and was thrown through the windshield. You are certain that the patient is dead. The patient's wife, who was driving the car, insists that you do something to save her husband. In this instance, you should:

    A. try to resuscitate the patient but stop after 5 minutes if there is no response.

    B. call medical control for instructions.

    C. pronounce the patient dead at the scene.

    D. initiate full resuscitation.

11. Your most appropriate course of action when confronted with a sudden death crisis is to:

    A. try to hide any unpleasant facts from the patient's family until the patient arrives at the hospital.

    B. answer questions as truthfully as possible and admit when you are unable to answer a question.

    C. help family members to avoid denying that a death has occurred.

    D. express your own feelings about the death to the family.

12. The protocol used by law enforcement agencies to collect and preserve evidence of a crime is called:

    A. crime scene management.

    B. crime victim management.

    C. evidence management.

    D. the chain of evidence.

Crisis Intervention

13. What condition occurs when certain abuses prevent a child from gaining weight or growing properly?

    A. Failure to thrive

    B. Emotional neglect

    C. Emotional withdrawal

    D. Emotional abandonment

14. You are called to a house where a 6-year-old boy may have a broken arm. The child's father tells you that his son fell down a flight of stairs. While you are examining the child, you notice some old burns and bruises on his skin. The boy seems withdrawn and does not respond when you ask him how he was hurt. What should you do?

    A. You should assume that the child is in too much pain to respond and question the father instead.

    B. You should tactfully lecture the father about child abuse and remove the child from the scene.

    C. You should remove the child from the scene with or without the father's consent and call law enforcement officials.

    D. You should remove the child from the scene with the father's consent and report a case of suspected child abuse to medical control.

15. Appropriate care for a patient who has attempted suicide should include:

    A. staying with the patient to ensure he or she does not make another attempt.

    B. leaving the patient in privacy while you discuss with the family the reasons for the attempt.

    C. staying with the patient while you discuss with the family the reasons for the attempt.

    D. trying to determine whether it was a serious attempt.

16. The first step in handling a SIDS crisis is to:

    A. console the parents.

    B. call law enforcement officials immediately.

    C. focus your attention on the infant.

    D. tell the family everything will be all right.

Chapter 23

17. The Critical Incident Stress Debriefing (CISD) program is designed to help:

    A. families deal with the sudden death of a loved one.

    B. law enforcement officials interview victims of a crime.

    C. law enforcement officials interview witnesses to a crime.

    D. emergency medical personnel cope with psychological reactions to job-related stresses.

18. You are at the scene of a serious automobile accident where one of the passengers has been decapitated. Your partner takes one look at the scene, turns pale, jokes that this patient "really lost his head," and announces that he cannot take anymore and is leaving the scene. You should recognize that your partner's statement is:

    A. a normal reaction to stress.

    B. an attempt to relax the patient's family.

    C. an attempt to describe the mechanism of injury.

    D. an appropriate description of the incident to give to medical control.

19. You are called to the home of a man who is terminally ill. He is conscious and alert, but is experiencing hypotension and bradycardia. His wife wants him to die in peace at home, but his son wants him to be transported to the hospital. The appropriate course of action is to:

    A. ask the patient what he wants and transport him only if he consents.

    B. ask the wife if the patient has a living will and abide by that.

    C. follow the instructions of the patient's wife.

    D. follow the instructions of the patient's son.

20. You are a witness to a patient's dying declaration. What should you do?

    A. Ask law enforcement officials for advice.

    B. Advise the patient's lawyer.

    C. Keep the declaration in confidence.

    D. Write down the statement word for word.

Crisis Intervention

21. Your care for a victim of assault should include:

    A. allowing the patient to ventilate anger.

    B. restraining the patient if emergency medical treatment is refused.

    C. assuming the patient has more serious physical injuries than emotional injuries.

    D. allowing law enforcement officials to question the patient before you begin treatment.

22. Decapitation occurs when:

    A. the patient has bled to death.

    B. the patient's head has been cut off.

    C. blood has pooled in the parts of the body closest to the ground.

    D. the patient's entire body has stiffened several hours after death.

23. You suspect that an automobile accident was a suicide attempt. Your primary responsibility in this situation is to:

    A. interview the family to find out why the attempt was made.

    B. tell law enforcement officials so they can question the family.

    C. discuss your suspicions with medical control and hospital personnel.

    D. collect any evidence available at the scene and transport smaller items with the patient.

24. Patients who attempt suicide by cutting their wrists may:

    A. survive because the blood vessels involved are not that large.

    B. not seek assistance from EMS because their will to die is so strong.

    C. bleed to death since the radial artery is so close to the skin surface.

    D. not survive because they almost always take an overdose of sedatives also.

Chapter 23

Answers

1: **C.** Only a licensed physician can legally pronounce a patient dead. (ECTSI 5, p. 656)

2: **A.** Lividity is a conclusive sign of death that occurs when dependent body parts turn bluish-red or purple due to blood settling to the lower parts of the body. (ECTSI 5, pp. 78–79, 656)

3: **B.** Rigor mortis is a conclusive sign of death that occurs when the entire body stiffens several hours after death. (ECTSI 5, pp. 78–79, 656)

4: **D.** Denial, anger, depression, and acceptance are the four phases of emotional response that a patient with a terminal illness usually experiences. (ECTSI 5, p. 657)

5: **D.** A dying declaration is a statement made by a patient who knows he is dying. It may be accepted as a legal document in a court of law in most states. (ECTSI 5, p. 658)

6: **B.** You should avoid examining the genitalia in a patient who has been raped, unless there is obvious bleeding that must be treated. (ECTSI 5, p. 661)

7: **A.** You will not be able to distinguish the difference between a gesture for help by a patient and a serious suicide attempt. (ECTSI 5, p. 664)

8: **C.** The first step in treating a victim of suspected child abuse is to remove the child from the environment producing the abuse. (ECTSI 5, pp. 568–569, 663)

9: **B.** Sudden infant death syndrome (SIDS) usually occurs in infants between 2 to 4 months of age. (ECTSI 5, pp. 568, 665)

10: **D.** When you are certain that a patient is dead, but the patient's family feels that something must be done to try to save the patient, you should initiate full resuscitation. You must understand, however, that once you begin you cannot stop until directed by a physician. (ECTSI 5, pp. 112–113, 656)

11: **B.** When faced with a sudden death crisis, answer questions as truthfully as possible and admit when you do not know an answer to a question. (ECTSI 5, pp. 656–657)

Crisis Intervention

12: **D.** The chain of evidence is the protocol used by law enforcement agencies to collect and preserve evidence of a crime. (ECTSI 5, p. 660)

13: **A.** When certain abuses prevent a child from gaining weight or growing properly it is called failure to thrive. (ECTSI 5, p. 662)

14: **D.** You are legally required to report any instance of suspected child abuse to the proper authorities. When you are treating a child you suspect has been abused, you should try to remove the child from the scene of the abuse, but you must have the parent's or guardian's consent to do so. In this case, the most appropriate course of action would be to try to get the father's permission to take the boy to the hospital and then call medical control to report your suspicions. (ECTSI 5, p. 663)

15: **A.** A patient who has attempted suicide should not be left alone because the patient might try again. (ECTSI 5, p. 664)

16: **C.** In a SIDS crisis, you should first focus your attention on the infant, in the event that he or she can be revived. (ECTSI 5, pp. 568, 665)

17: **D.** The Critical Incident Stress Debriefing (CISD) program is designed to help emergency medical personnel cope with psychological reactions to job-related stresses. (ECTSI 5, pp. 666–667)

18: **A.** In this case, you should recognize that your partner is responding to a very stressful situation. You should remind him to try to maintain a calm, professional manner in this situation. (ECTSI 5, p. 666)

19: **A.** When you are faced with one family member who wishes that a terminally ill patient be left at home to die and another who wishes the patient to be taken to the hospital, you should ask the patient about his wishes, if possible, and transport him only if he consents. (ECTSI 5, p. 658)

20: **D.** You should write down a patient's dying declaration word for word because in some states it may be used as a sworn statement in a court of law. (ECTSI 5, p. 658)

21: **A.** A patient who has been assaulted should be encouraged to talk in order to ventilate the anger that is often a reaction to a stressful situation. (ECTSI 5, p. 659)

22: **B.** Decapitation is a conclusive sign of death that occurs when a patient's head has been cut off. (ECTSI 5, pp. 654, 656)

Chapter 23

23: **C.** In this situation, you should discuss your suspicions with medical control and hospital personnel. (ECTSI 5, p. 664)

24: **A.** Many patients who cut their wrists in a suicide attempt do not bleed to death because the blood vessels involved are not that large. (ECTSI 5, p. 664)

Chapter 24

Handling and Packaging the Patient

Chapter Goals

The exercises in this chapter are designed to help the student to:

- describe the basic methods for lifting and handling patients.

- explain how to use an ambulance stretcher.

- describe different situations in which a rescuer may need to lift and move patients.

- explain different patient packaging techniques.

Chapter 24

Multiple-Choice Questions

Select the correct answer for each of the following questions. Each question has only *one* correct or best answer.

1. Which of the following methods would be most appropriate for a lone rescuer to remove a patient from the vicinity of a possible explosion?

    A. Log roll

    B. Clothes drag

    C. Seat lift and carry

    D. Extremity lift and carry

2. When lifting a stretcher, you should:

    A. bend your hips, knees, back, and arms.

    B. bend at the waist and keep your back straight.

    C. place your hands palm up under the litter.

    D. lift with a smooth straightening of your legs.

3. When you plan to use a chair to carry a patient down a flight of stairs, you must first test the chair for sturdiness, and then:

    A. tilt the chair backwards.

    B. speak clearly to the patient.

    C. be sure the patient is well secured.

    D. be sure the patient's hands are in his or her lap.

4. If a patient is injured, but is not in immediate danger from fire or building collapse, you should first direct your attention to the:

    A. patient's level of consciousness.

    B. patient's airway, breathing, and circulation.

    C. equipment you will need for extrication.

    D. number of people you will need for assistance.

Handling and Packaging the Patient

5. Of the following, which is the most efficient way to transfer a patient from a bed to a stretcher?

   A. Drawsheet method

   B. Pack-strap carry

   C. 2-person seat carry

   D. 2-person pickup

6. What type of stretcher should be used to move a patient with a suspected spinal injury from a height of 15'?

   A. Split-frame

   B. Ambulance

   C. Stokes

   D. Scoop

7. When using a split-frame stretcher to move a patient, you must make sure to:

   A. avoid "scooping" the patient onto the stretcher.

   B. carry the loaded stretcher at a 45° angle.

   C. slip the stretcher under the long axis of the patient's body.

   D. leave both sides of the patient's body accessible.

8. In what position should an unconscious patient be transported on a stretcher?

   A. Prone

   B. Lateral

   C. Supine

   D. Semisitting

Chapter 24

9. To safely transport a patient down a steep flight of stairs, you should use either a:

    A. split-frame stretcher or stair chair.

    B. split-frame stretcher or full backboard.

    C. stair chair or full backboard.

    D. stair chair or knockdown stretcher.

10. Which of the following transport devices is adequate for standard spinal injury immobilization?

    A. Scoop stretcher

    B. Backboard

    C. Stair chair

    D. Ambulance stretcher

11. You are called to a house where a conscious, alert man may be experiencing angina. The patient is lying in his bedroom on the second floor. The most appropriate way to transport this patient to the ambulance is to:

    A. help the patient walk down the stairs.

    B. place the patient in a stair chair and then carry him down.

    C. place the patient in a Stokes litter and then lower him from the window.

    D. carry the patient down the stairs with your partner, using the extremity lift and carry.

12. The log roll is a technique used to:

    A. place a patient on a backboard.

    B. place a patient into an ambulance.

    C. transport a patient safely.

    D. splint a patient effectively.

Handling and Packaging the Patient

13. How many rescuers are needed to perform a log roll if the patient has a suspected spinal injury?

    A. 2

    B. 3

    C. 4

    D. 5

14. When transporting a child, you should remember to carry an extra blanket because children tend to:

    A. need extra support under the neck.

    B. lose body heat more rapidly than adults.

    C. become frantic, and the blanket should be used to hide their eyes.

    D. become violent, and the blanket will have a calming effect.

15. Moving a patient in a stretcher up a hill may involve:

    A. multiple-person stretcher passes.

    B. walking uphill sideways with both hands on the basket.

    C. walking uphill while supporting the stretcher with one hand.

    D. walking uphill while supporting the stretcher on the rescuers' shoulders.

16. An injured patient who needs to be moved to safety quickly because of a potential building collapse should be:

    A. removed using the one-person walking assist.

    B. pulled along the long axis of the body.

    C. loaded onto a knockdown stretcher.

    D. secured to a backboard.

Chapter 24

17. A short spine board should be placed beneath the mattress at the head of the stretcher in the event that:

    A. CPR needs to be performed.

    B. the front wheels of the stretcher collapse.

    C. the patient must be restrained.

    D. transport over rough ground is necessary.

18. When using a split-frame stretcher, in order to place the stretcher under the patient, you must separate:

    A. both halves.

    B. only the foot end.

    C. only the head end.

    D. the middle section from the body.

19. A patient receiving supplemental oxygen is sitting upright in a wheelchair and must be carried down six stairs. The wheelchair should be carried downstairs by how many EMTs?

    A. 2, with a watcher

    B. 3

    C. 4

    D. 4, with a watcher

20. A patient secured to a split-frame stretcher should be carried down a flight of stairs:

    A. by at least four EMTs.

    B. tilted to one side.

    C. head first.

    D. feet first.

270 Student Review Manual

Handling and Packaging the Patient

21. To avoid injuring yourself while lifting a patient, you should:

    A. lift using your legs.

    B. lift using your back.

    C. only use one hand.

    D. always use both hands.

22. A patient immobilized on a backboard can be placed in the shock position by:

    A. raising the arms above the head.

    B. placing the patient on his or her side.

    C. elevating the legs.

    D. elevating the head.

23. A patient's respirations may be affected after being placed in a Trendelenburg's position because:

    A. blood rushes from the head when the head is higher than the heart.

    B. abdominal organs may press against the diaphragm.

    C. the patient's knees are flexed.

    D. the patient is in a side-lying position.

24. The process of transferring, positioning, and securing an ill or injured patient to a stretcher or other carrying device is known as:

    A. packaging.

    B. handling.

    C. preparing.

    D. triage.

Chapter 24

25. During initial care in the field, the objective of every patient-handling situation is to:

   A. use universal precautions.

   B. give the patient the most complete care possible.

   C. remove the patient from the scene as quickly as possible.

   D. ensure that additional injury is not sustained by the patient or the rescuer.

Answers

1: **B.** If you had to act alone to remove a patient from the vicinity of a possible explosion, you would use a clothes drag, pulling with the long axis of the patient's body. Other one-person rescue methods are the blanket drag and the firefighter's drag. (ECTSI 5, p. 678)

2: **D.** When lifting a stretcher, you should lift with a smooth straightening of your legs. (ECTSI 5, pp. 688–689)

3: **C.** When using a chair to carry a patient down stairs, you must first test it for sturdiness and then make sure the patient is well secured in the chair. (ECTSI 5, p. 692)

4: **B.** If a patient is injured, but is not in immediate danger from fire or building collapse, your attention should first be directed to the patient's airway, breathing, and circulation. (ECTSI 5, p. 671)

5: **A.** An efficient method to use when transferring a patient from a bed to a stretcher is the drawsheet method. (ECTSI 5, p. 686)

6: **C.** A patient with a suspected spinal injury should be evacuated from a height using horizontal lowering of a Stokes stretcher. (ECTSI 5, p. 731)

7: **D.** If you use a split-frame stretcher to move a patient, you must make sure that both sides of the patient's body are accessible. (ECTSI 5, p. 692)

8: **B.** An unconscious person should be transported on a stretcher in a lateral position. (ECTSI 5, p. 690)

9: **A.** Use of either a stair chair or split-frame stretcher is effective for moving a patient down a narrow flight of stairs. (ECTSI 5, p. 692)

Handling and Packaging the Patient

10: **B.** Of the choices listed, only the backboard provides adequate support for spinal immobilization. The ambulance stretcher requires the addition of a short spine board. (ECTSI 5, p. 692)

11: **B.** A conscious patient with possible angina should be carried (not walked) from an upstairs bedroom to the ambulance in a stair chair. The stair chair keeps pressure off the chest, unlike the extremity lift and carry. The Stokes would be appropriate if the patient had spinal injuries. (ECTSI 5, pp. 449, 681, 692, 730)

12: **A.** The log roll is a technique used to place a patient on a backboard. (ECTSI 5, p. 684)

13: **C.** Four rescuers are needed to perform a log roll if a patient has a suspected spinal injury. (ECTSI 5, p. 684)

14: **B.** Children tend to lose body heat rapidly due to their relatively larger body surface area. This means that the younger the child, the more rapidly you should cover the child as a protection against the elements. (ECTSI 5, p. 674)

15: **A.** Rescues in rough or hilly terrain may involve using multiple-person stretcher passes. (ECTSI 5, p. 727)

16: **B.** An injured patient who must be moved to safety quickly because of a possible building collapse, should be pulled along the long axis of the body. (ECTSI 5, p. 678)

17: **A.** A short spine board should be placed beneath the mattress at the head of the stretcher in the event that CPR needs to be performed. (ECTSI 5, p. 685)

18: **A.** You must separate both halves before placing the patient on a split-frame stretcher. (ECTSI 5, p. 693)

19: **A.** A patient who is being carried down a flight of stairs in a wheelchair must be carried by at least two EMTs, with a watcher for additional safety. (ECTSI 5, p. 692)

20: **D.** A patient who is secured to a split-frame stretcher should be carried down stairs feet first. (ECTSI 5, p. 689)

21: **A.** You should lift a patient using your legs in order to avoid injuring yourself. (ECTSI 5, p. 676)

Chapter 24

22: **C.** A patient who has been immobilized on a backboard can be placed in the shock position by elevating the patient's legs. (ECTSI 5, pp. 213, 868)

23: **B.** A patient's respirations may be affected after being placed in a Trendelenburg's position because abdominal organs may press against the diaphragm. (ECTSI 5, pp. 213, 868)

24: **A.** Packaging is the term used for transferring, positioning, and strapping a patient to a stretcher or other carrying device. (ECTSI 5, p. 672)

25: **D.** Ensuring that additional injury is not sustained by the patient or rescuer is the objective of every patient-handling situation in its initial stages. (ECTSI 5, p. 673)

Chapter 25

Ambulance Operations

Chapter Goals

The exercises in this chapter are designed to help the student to:

- discuss the defensive driving techniques necessary when driving the ambulance.

- describe appropriate approaching and parking procedures at the scene of an automobile accident.

- explain why it is necessary to stop momentarily before proceeding through an intersection with a red light, even with lights and siren running.

- identify factors that contribute to the problem of excessive speed in driving the ambulance.

- describe the qualifications needed to be an emergency vehicle driver.

Chapter 25

Multiple-Choice Questions

Select the correct answer for each of the following questions. Each question has only *one* correct or best answer.

1. The primary objective of the emergency vehicle driver is to:

    A. act as a chauffeur so the patient can be treated in the hospital.

    B. get the patient to the hospital in a safe and efficient manner.

    C. get the patient to the hospital as quickly as possible.

    D. clear traffic using flashing lights and sirens.

2. Which of the following statements about using right-of-way privileges is true?

    A. The ambulance is allowed by federal law to proceed through any intersection without stopping.

    B. An ambulance with its lights and siren running is allowed by federal law to proceed through any intersection.

    C. Each state has the same law regarding right-of-way privileges.

    D. Each state may have a slightly different law regarding right-of-way privileges.

3. A traffic light turns red as the ambulance on an urgent call is approaching an intersection. There are no vehicles in front of the ambulance. You should:

    A. stop, sound the siren if necessary, and proceed when safe.

    B. sound the siren, maintain speed, and proceed.

    C. bypass the traffic light by turning into a side street.

    D. turn off the lights and siren and wait for the light to change.

4. When following another vehicle in the same lane, the ambulance should remain at least how many seconds behind that vehicle?

    A. 2

    B. 3

    C. 4

    D. 10

Ambulance Operations

5. An ambulance may cross a double yellow line into the opposite lane only when:

    A. any upcoming traffic signals are green.

    B. the road is straight and flat, even if there is heavy traffic.

    C. the driver has a clear and unobstructed view of the road.

    D. the lights and siren are running, even if other cars have not pulled over.

6. At the time of dispatch, the emergency vehicle driver should:

    A. try to follow the "normal" route, even during rush hour.

    B. select the shortest and least congested route to the scene.

    C. use the siren and flashing lights to ensure safe passage.

    D. travel on as many one-way streets as possible.

7. After each trip, the emergency vehicle driver must make a run inspection, which includes:

    A. cleaning and decontaminating the interior of the ambulance.

    B. writing a report of all that occurred during the run.

    C. changing the oil and filter.

    D. checking wheel alignment.

8. When traveling on a multi-lane highway, the emergency vehicle driver should try to keep to the:

    A. extreme right lane, so other motorists can move over to the left.

    B. extreme left lane, so other motorists can move over to the right.

    C. center lane, so traffic can flow smoothly around the ambulance.

    D. right shoulder, so traffic flow is not disrupted.

Chapter 25

9. You have been called to the scene of an automobile accident that occurred on a hill. You should park the ambulance:

    A. uphill of the accident site on the same side of the street.

    B. uphill of the accident site on the opposite side of the street.

    C. downhill of the accident site on the same side of the street.

    D. downhill of the accident site on the opposite side of the street.

10. To avoid hitting another vehicle while driving an ambulance in traffic, you should:

    A. turn on the lights and siren so the other vehicle will know you are there.

    B. try to maintain an open space in an adjacent lane as an escape route.

    C. speed up quickly to move around the other vehicle.

    D. brake hard to stop the ambulance.

11. If using the siren during transport disturbs the patient, and it is not absolutely necessary to use it, you should:

    A. disregard the patient's feelings because the law requires the use of lights and siren.

    B. turn it off and adjust your driving accordingly.

    C. use the yelp or hi-lo instead.

    D. use the air horn instead.

12. Determining the best route to the scene at the time of dispatch is:

    A. called defensive driving.

    B. called the 4-second rule.

    C. part of the run inspection.

    D. a general guideline for safe driving.

Ambulance Operations

13. One of the factors that contributes to the problem of excessive use of vehicle speed during an emergency call is:

    A. the driver's lack of training in an ambulance's safe operation.

    B. an experienced dispatcher's advice to use speed over safety.

    C. the chassis set of the ambulance.

    D. the coefficient of friction.

14. In what positions on the steering wheel should your hands be when driving an ambulance?

    A. Twelve o'clock and six o'clock

    B. Eleven o'clock and one o'clock

    C. Nine o'clock and three o'clock

    D. Eight o'clock and four o'clock

15. Use of a police escort may be a dangerous practice in an intersection because:

    A. bystanders could gather to watch and cause traffic problems.

    B. too many emergency vehicles with sirens and lights could cause motorists to panic.

    C. trying to move two emergency vehicles through congested traffic is more difficult than one and may take too much time.

    D. a motorist seeing the police car pass might assume it is the only emergency vehicle and could proceed, hitting the ambulance.

16. A serious hazard for an ambulance driving through an intersection where a green light is about to turn red is the possibility that:

    A. another motorist may be timing the red light to avoid stopping and will proceed into the intersection.

    B. the ambulance may hydroplane on the pavement if it does not slow down.

    C. the ambulance may not corner efficiently if it does not slow down.

    D. right-of-way privileges may be abused.

Chapter 25

17. What are the most common and usually most serious hazards that occur when driving an ambulance?

    A. Rollover accidents

    B. Intersection accidents

    C. Loss of braking ability

    D. Hydroplaning incidents

18. Training requirements for an EMT who drives an ambulance are:

    A. similar to those for other EMTs, but also include some legal courses.

    B. totally different from those for other EMTs.

    C. less stringent than those for other EMTs.

    D. the same as those for other EMTs.

Answers

1: **B.** The driver of an emergency vehicle must try to get the patient to the hospital in a safe and efficient manner. (ECTSI 5, p. 749)

2: **D.** Each state may have a slightly different law regarding right-of-way privileges. (ECTSI 5, p. 754)

3: **A.** When the ambulance approaches a red light at an intersection and there is no traffic in front of it, the driver should stop at the light, sound the siren, and proceed when certain that the intersection is clear. (ECTSI 5, pp. 754–755)

4: **C.** When following another vehicle in the same lane, you should stay at least 4 seconds behind the other vehicle. This is known as the "4-second rule." (ECTSI 5, p. 756)

5: **C.** An ambulance may cross a double yellow line into the opposite lane only when the driver has a clear and unobstructed view of the road. (ECTSI 5, p. 756)

6: **B.** At the time of dispatch, the emergency vehicle driver should select the shortest and least congested route to the scene. (ECTSI 5, p. 755)

Ambulance Operations

7: **A.** As part of the run inspection after each trip, the emergency vehicle driver should make certain the interior of the ambulance is cleaned and decontaminated. (ECTSI 5, p. 758)

8: **B.** When traveling on a multi-lane highway, the emergency vehicle driver should keep to the extreme left because there is less traffic under most conditions. It also allows other motorists to move to the right in a normal manner. (ECTSI 5, p. 754)

9: **A.** When responding to an accident that has taken place on a hill, the ambulance should be parked uphill of the accident on the same side of the street. (ECTSI 5, p. 756)

10: **B.** To avoid hitting another vehicle while driving an ambulance in traffic, you should always try to maintain an open space in an adjacent lane as an escape route. (ECTSI 5, p. 756)

11: **B.** If using the siren during transport disturbs the patient, and use of the siren is not absolutely necessary, you should turn off the siren and adjust your driving accordingly. (ECTSI 5, p. 755)

12: **D.** One of the general guidelines for safe operation of an ambulance is determining the best route to the scene at the time of dispatch. (ECTSI 5, p. 755)

13: **A.** One of the factors that may contribute to the problem of excessive use of speed during a response to an emergency call is the driver's lack of training in an ambulance's safe operation. (ECTSI 5, p. 750)

14: **C.** Your hands should be placed at the nine o'clock and three o'clock positions on the steering wheel when you are driving an ambulance. (ECTSI 5, p. 750)

15: **D.** Use of a police escort may be dangerous in an intersection because a motorist hearing a siren and seeing the police car pass may assume that only one emergency vehicle is passing. The motorist may then proceed into the intersection and possibly hit the ambulance. (ECTSI 5, p. 754)

16: **A.** An ambulance driving through an intersection where a green light is about to turn red faces a serious hazard from an intersecting motorist who may be timing the lights to avoid stopping at the intersection. The motorist may know his or her red light will be turning green and will proceed into the intersection, hitting the ambulance. (ECTSI 5, p. 755)

Chapter 25

17: **B.** Accidents that occur in intersections are the most common and usually most serious hazards that occur when driving an ambulance. (ECTSI 5, p. 754)

18: **D.** Training requirements for the EMT who drives the ambulance are the same as those for any other EMT. (ECTSI 5, p. 756)

Chapter 26

Intravenous Therapy

Chapter Goals

The exercises in this chapter are designed to help the student to:

- identify the equipment and supplies needed for IV therapy.

- describe the steps in starting an IV line.

- explain why monitoring of the patient and the IV is necessary.

- describe possible complications of IV therapy.

- identify indications for IV therapy.

- calculate the appropriate drip rate for various IV administration sets.

Chapter 26

Multiple-Choice Questions

Select the correct answer for each of the following questions. Each question has only *one* correct or best answer.

1. IV volume replacement would **NOT** be indicated for which of the following conditions?

    A. Severe burns

    B. Acute pulmonary edema

    C. Dehydration

    D. Gastrointestinal bleeding

2. Connecting and starting an IV line in a patient without first flushing the administration set can result in:

    A. an infection.

    B. severe diarrhea.

    C. an air embolism.

    D. a pyrogenic reaction.

3. Of the following, which intervention would be considered an invasive procedure?

    A. Inflation of a pneumatic antishock garment (PASG)

    B. Administration of high-flow oxygen

    C. Application of a tourniquet

    D. Initiation of an IV line

4. What is the abbreviation for an IV solution containing 5% dextrose?

    A. FPD5

    B. D5W

    C. D5S

    D. WD5

Intravenous Therapy

5. An IV with normal saline solution contains how much sodium?

    A. 0.9%

    B. 2.5%

    C. 50%

    D. 75%

6. Insertion of a catheter into a vein to administer fluids or medications is referred to as:

    A. phlebotomy.

    B. dialysis.

    C. IV therapy.

    D. gastric lavage.

7. Normal saline solution does **NOT** come in which of the following preparations?

    A. 1/8 NS

    B. 1/4 NS

    C. 1/2 NS

    D. NS

8. Of the following, which IV solution is the most commonly used in a prehospital setting?

    A. Sodium chloride

    B. Potassium

    C. Calcium

    D. Glucose

Chapter 26

9. Which of the following preparations is a colloid IV solution made up of large molecules of dextrose?

    A. Dextroflow

    B. Dextran

    C. Dexacol

    D. Dexatrim

10. Which of the following statements about IV crystalloid solutions is **FALSE**?

    A. They can carry oxygen.

    B. They can carry medications.

    C. They can replace essential electrolytes.

    D. They can be infused to increase blood pressure.

11. Which of the following supplies is **NOT** necessary to have on hand to initiate an IV line?

    A. 50-mL syringe

    B. Prep swabs

    C. Tourniquet

    D. Administration set

12. Which of the following is **NOT** a necessary step before starting an IV?

    A. Applying a tourniquet

    B. Explaining the procedure to the patient

    C. Confirming that the vein has a pulse

    D. Assembling the necessary equipment

Intravenous Therapy

13. What is the first, most important consideration in selecting a solution for an IV infusion?

    A. Confirm that you have selected the correct solution.

    B. Make sure that the sterile seals on the bag of fluid are intact.

    C. Examine the solution to make sure that it is clear.

    D. Make sure that the expiration date has not passed.

14. What type of IV administration set is designed to keep an IV line open with a minimal volume infusion?

    A. Mini-drip set

    B. Slow-flow set

    C. Volume set

    D. Solution set

15. What type of IV administration set is capable of providing large amounts of fluid in a short period of time?

    A. Mini-drip set

    B. Slow-flow set

    C. Volume set

    D. Solution set

16. Special large-bore trauma infusion tubing may enable the administration of up to how many liters of solution per minute?

    A. 1

    B. 2

    C. 3

    D. 4

Chapter 26

17. EMTs generally use what two types of IV needles or catheters?

    A. Catheter over the needle or butterfly

    B. Catheter over the needle or J-wire set

    C. Catheter through the needle or butterfly

    D. Catheter through the needle or plain steel

18. After the administration set is attached to the IV bag, you should prepare the drip chamber by holding the bag:

    A. lower than the drip chamber, then squeezing and releasing the drip chamber until it is half full.

    B. lower than the drip chamber, then squeezing and releasing the drip chamber until it is full.

    C. higher than the drip chamber, then squeezing and releasing the drip chamber until it is half full.

    D. higher than the drip chamber, then squeezing and releasing the drip chamber until it is full.

19. Which of the following statements about IV needles and catheters is **FALSE**?

    A. IV needles and catheters are sized according to gauge.

    B. A large-diameter IV needle will have a small gauge number.

    C. A small-diameter IV needle will have a small gauge number.

    D. The larger the internal diameter, the more fluid can be infused.

20. What gauge of catheter should be used on a patient who requires large volumes of IV infusion?

    A. 4 to 8

    B. 14 to 18

    C. 20 to 22

    D. 26 to 28

Intravenous Therapy

21. Before starting an IV line, you should ask the patient about allergies to which of the following substances?

    A. Iodine

    B. Blood

    C. Salt

    D. Dust

22. Which of the following sites would be a poor choice to attempt an IV insertion?

    A. Left dorsal hand

    B. In a burned extremity

    C. Antecubital fossa

    D. Right forearm

23. An IV tourniquet should be placed at approximately what location in relation to the venipuncture site?

    A. 1" to 2" proximal to the site

    B. 2" to 4" distal to the site

    C. 4" to 6" distal to the site

    D. 6" to 8" proximal to the site

24. The IV constricting band or tourniquet should be placed tight enough to restrict:

    A. either type of blood flow.

    B. both venous and arterial blood flow.

    C. venous blood flow but not arterial blood flow.

    D. arterial blood flow but not venous blood flow.

Chapter 26

25. You receive an order to infuse fluid at 20 mL/h. If the administration set delivers 60 drops per mL, the flow rate would be how many drops per minute? (Note: 1 mL = 1 cc)

    A. 50 gtts/min

    B. 40 gtts/min

    C. 30 gtts/min

    D. 20 gtts/min

26. You receive an order to infuse fluid at 10 mL/min. If the administration set delivers 17 drops per mL, the flow rate would be how many drops per minute? (Note: 1 mL = 1 cc)

    A. 2.8 gtts/min

    B. 10 gtts/min

    C. 102 gtts/min

    D. 170 gtts/min

27. You receive an order to infuse fluid at 4 mL/min. If the administration set delivers 10 drops per mL, the flow rate would be how many drops per minute? (Note: 1 mL = 1 cc)

    A. 0.66 gtts/min

    B. 40 gtts/min

    C. 100 gtts/min

    D. 240 gtts/min

28. Which of the following words best describes the goal of preparing a site for the initiation of an IV line?

    A. Disinfect

    B. Wipe

    C. Scrub

    D. Clean

Intravenous Therapy

29. Which of the following prep swabs should be used to prepare an IV site?

    A. Povoiodine and alcohol

    B. Dextrose and povoiodine

    C. Alcohol and soap

    D. Soap and water

30. Which of the following IV fluids contains sodium chloride, calcium chloride, and potassium chloride?

    A. D5W

    B. 1/2 NS

    C. Normal saline solution

    D. Lactated Ringer's solution

31. Before you perform the venipuncture, you should prepare to insert the IV needle at an angle of:

    A. 10°, with the bevel up.

    B. 20°, with the bevel down.

    C. 30°, with the bevel up.

    D. 40°, with the bevel down.

32. As the needle first enters the vein, you should anticipate:

    A. a flash back of blood at the needle hub.

    B. a clicking sound and resistance at the needle hub.

    C. a whistling sound as air rushes through the tubing.

    D. nothing at all, except perhaps the patient's cry of pain.

Chapter 26

33. What potentially serious complication can occur if an IV needle is removed from the catheter and then reinserted?

    A. Circulatory overload

    B. Catheter shear

    C. Hypertensive crisis

    D. Cardiovascular collapse

34. Infusion of IV fluid into surrounding tissues rather than into the vein is called:

    A. infiltration.

    B. embolism.

    C. infection.

    D. catheterization.

35. A butterfly needle that is accidentally manipulated or moved from side to side after it is in the vein may cause:

    A. epileptic seizures.

    B. the vein to be cut.

    C. fluid overload.

    D. air embolism.

36. Which of the following is **NOT** a sign of overhydration or circulatory overload?

    A. Rales

    B. Dyspnea

    C. Orthostatic hypotension

    D. Distention of the neck veins

Intravenous Therapy

37. After cannulating a vein, you remove the needle, connect the administration set, and hang the IV bag from the ceiling hook in the ambulance. You now notice blood pulsating back up into the tubing. Which of the following has likely occurred?

    A. The administration set is faulty.

    B. The patient has atherosclerosis.

    C. The IV bag contains the wrong solution.

    D. An artery has been cannulated.

38. What is the most common problem at the site of a failed IV attempt?

    A. Total catheter shear

    B. Formation of a hematoma

    C. Development of severe itching and rash

    D. Development of septic shock within 24 hours

39. You believe that you have inadvertently cannulated an artery in your attempt to start an IV. The most appropriate course of action would be to:

    A. open the administration set until it is wide open.

    B. wait for the bleeding to stop on its own.

    C. remove the catheter and apply direct pressure to the site.

    D. place the IV bag into a pressure infusor and pump it up.

40. Which of the following is a late complication of IV therapy that is not ordinarily seen by EMTs in the field?

    A. Thrombophlebitis

    B. Local infiltration

    C. Tape at the site comes loose

    D. Formation of a hematoma

Chapter 26

41. You start a large-bore IV line at a wide-open rate on a patient with congestive heart failure. Approximately 10 minutes after the line is started, the patient is unconscious, cyanotic, and sweating profusely. Your care of the patient should now focus on treating:

    A. fluid overload.

    B. an air embolism.

    C. a severe infection.

    D. an arterial puncture.

42. While rare, some patients may have an anaphylactic reaction to IV therapy. The reaction usually occurs because:

    A. too much fluid is infused intravenously.

    B. the person who started the IV did not wear gloves.

    C. the patient is allergic to the medication being administered.

    D. normal saline solution is infused instead of lactated Ringer's solution.

43. You are preparing to transport a patient who has had an IV line started in his right hand. The hospital is over an hour away. Twenty minutes later you are assessing the patient and see swelling and some redness around the IV site. The skin around the IV needle is warm to touch. The appropriate course of action would be to:

    A. place an ice pack on the site.

    B. place a constricting band above the site.

    C. change the IV line to the left hand.

    D. leave the IV in place until you reach the hospital.

44. Continued pain or burning at an IV site is most likely a sign of:

    A. infiltration.

    B. fluid overload.

    C. an air embolism.

    D. hypotension.

Intravenous Therapy

45. The introduction of whole blood or blood products into the vascular system is called:

    A. an infusion.

    B. a phlebotomy.

    C. a transfusion.

    D. a venipuncture.

46. Which of the following is **NOT** a skill of an EMT-A?

    A. Monitoring a patient's blood pressure

    B. Initiating IV fluid therapy

    C. Splinting a fractured extremity

    D. Controlling bleeding with direct pressure

47. The introduction of fluid other than blood or blood products into the vascular system is called:

    A. an infusion.

    B. a phlebotomy.

    C. a transfusion.

    D. a venipuncture.

48. Which of the following factors would **NOT** cause an IV to stop running?

    A. The patient's elbow is bent.

    B. There is a kink in the tubing.

    C. The IV bag is hung too high above the patient.

    D. The IV fluid has infiltrated into surrounding tissue.

Chapter 26

49. You must start an IV line in a patient who is entangled in farm equipment in the middle of a frozen farm field. In this cold environment, you should continually assess the patient for possible development of:

   A. a hematoma.

   B. a catheter shear.

   C. hypothermia.

   D. aphasia.

50. Which of the following conditions is **NOT** considered a systemic complication of IV therapy?

   A. Simple fainting

   B. Air embolism

   C. Circulatory overload

   D. Tissue sloughing

Answers

1: **B.** A patient with pulmonary edema is already overhydrated, so volume replacement would be contraindicated. If a patient with pulmonary edema has an IV line for medication administration, the IV line should be run at a TKO rate. (ECTSI 5, p. 783)

2: **C.** Even though the amount of air in the IV administration set and tubing appears small, an air embolism could still develop. The patient may rapidly lose consciousness, go into shock, and if left untreated, could possibly die. (ECTSI 5, p. 791)

3: **D.** Invasive procedures are those that involve placing medical devices or instruments into the body, such as IV therapy and intubation. (ECTSI 5, p. 783)

4: **B.** D5W is the correct abbreviation for an IV solution containing 5% dextrose. (ECTSI 5, p. 784)

5: **A.** Normal saline is a crystalloid isotonic solution and contains 0.9% sodium. (ECTSI 5, p. 784)

Intravenous Therapy

6: **C.** Placement of a catheter or needle into a vein to administer fluids or medication is called intravenous (IV) therapy. (ECTSI 5, p. 784)

7: **A.** One-half normal saline (1/2 NS), one-quarter normal saline (1/4 NS), and normal saline (NS) are all crystalloid solutions that contain sodium chloride and are commonly used for IV therapy. (ECTSI 5, p. 784)

8: **A.** While glucose is commonly used for IV infusion in the prehospital setting, it does not contain electrolytes. Preparations with sodium chloride contain electrolytes and are the most commonly used solutions in the prehospital setting. (ECTSI 5, p. 784)

9: **B.** Dextran is a colloid solution made up of large molecules of dextrose that are not metabolized; therefore, they remain in the vascular space far longer than crystalloid solutions. (ECTSI 5, p. 784)

10: **A.** Both colloid and crystalloid IV solutions can support blood pressure, replace electrolytes, and carry medications. However, they cannot carry oxygen as does hemoglobin. (ECTSI 5, p. 784)

11: **A.** Prep swabs, a tourniquet, and an administration set are absolutely necessary to start an IV line, whereas a 50-mL syringe is not. (ECTSI 5, p. 785)

12: **C.** Veins do not have a pulse, arteries do. Checking for a pulse before starting an IV line reduces the likelihood of cannulating an artery by mistake. (ECTSI 5, p. 787)

13: **A.** While all of the answer choices are important steps in selecting an IV solution, it is most important to first confirm that you have selected the correct solution for the patient. Checking the expiration date, the color of the solution, and that seals are intact should certainly be done before the solution is administered to the patient. (ECTSI 5, p. 785)

14: **A.** Mini-drip sets administer 1 mL (or cc) with every 60 drops that pass through the drip chamber. This makes mini-drip sets a fine choice when the purpose of the IV is to keep the vein open and to provide a route for medications, rather than provide volume replacement. (ECTSI 5, p. 785)

15: **D.** When large volumes of fluid need to be infused rapidly, a solution set, or maxi-set, is the administration set of choice. (ECTSI 5, p. 785)

16: **A.** When large-bore trauma infusion tubing is used, up to 1 liter a minute of fluid can be infused. (ECTSI 5, p. 785)

Chapter 26

17: **A.** EMTs most commonly use either the catheter over the needle or the butterfly (plain needle) device. (ECTSI 5, p. 786)

18: **C.** By holding the IV bag above the drip chamber, you can fill the chamber by squeezing the bag. The chamber should be no more than half full, so the drops are visible as they enter the chamber. This allows for accurate adjustment of the flow rate. (ECTSI 5, p. 786)

19: **C.** Of the answer choices listed, a small-diameter IV needle will have a small gauge number is a false statement. (ECTSI 5, p. 786)

20: **B.** To infuse large volumes of fluid in the prehospital setting, you should select a 14-, 16-, or 18-gauge catheter. Even though 12-gauge catheters are occasionally used, they are extremely difficult to insert in a peripheral vein due to the smaller internal diameter size of the vein in relation to the IV catheter. (ECTSI 5, p. 786)

21: **A.** Before starting an IV line, you should ask the patient about allergies to iodine, adhesive materials, and medications. Dust, blood, and salt allergies would not be pertinent in this situation. (ECTSI 5, p. 786)

22: **B.** Injured extremities are not ideal sites for the initiation of an IV line, particularly if the injury is a burn. With burn injuries, there is loss of fluid at the site. (ECTSI 5, p. 787)

23: **D.** Placing the IV tourniquet about 6" to 8" proximal to the site facilitates filling of the vein, yet it is far enough above the site that it will not be in the way of venipuncture. (ECTSI 5, p. 787)

24: **C.** The vein becomes engorged, and thus easier to enter, if venous return is restricted and the artery is allowed to flow. (ECTSI 5, p. 787)

25: **D.** To calculate the flow rate, multiply the amount of fluid to be infused by the drops/mL (or cc) for the drip chamber, and then divide this number by the time of infusion. In this situation, 20 mL is to be infused per hour by a 60-drop mini-set. The equation is as follows: (20 x 60) ÷ 60 = 20 gtts/min. (ECTSI 5, p. 790)

26: **D.** In this situation, 10 mL is to be infused per minute by a 17-drop drip chamber. The equation is as follows: (10 x 17) ÷ 1 = 170 gtts/min. (ECTSI 5, p. 790)

27: **B.** In this situation, 4 mL is to be infused per minute by a 10-drop drip chamber. The equation is as follows: (4 x 10) ÷ 1 = 40 gtts/min. (ECTSI 5, p. 790)

Intravenous Therapy

28: **A.** The goal when preparing an IV insertion site is to disinfect the site, and as a result, remove the potential for infection as much as possible. (ECTSI 5, p. 787)

29: **A.** Povoiodine is used to disinfect the site, and alcohol is used to remove the povoiodine. (ECTSI 5, p. 787)

30: **D.** Lactated Ringer's solution is an isotonic, balanced, buffered crystalloid solution that is used to replace lost blood volume and electrolytes. It contains sodium chloride, calcium chloride, and potassium chloride. (ECTSI 5, p. 784)

31: **C.** Entering the skin at an angle of 30° allows penetration without too much depth too quickly. The bevel should be up, which also helps to control the speed of entry. Increasing the angle of entry by turning the bevel down would most likely result in insertion through both sides of the vein, also known as " blowing the vein." (ECTSI 5, p. 788)

32: **A.** As the needle enters the vein, blood will "flash back" through the needle into the needle hub, confirming that the vein has been cannulated. (ECTSI 5, p. 788)

33: **B.** Once it has been removed, a needle should not be reinserted. Reinsertion may allow the needle to cut or shear off the end of the catheter, which would then begin to travel towards the heart and the right atrium, with potentially serious complications. (ECTSI 5, p. 788)

34: **A.** Infiltration is the proper term to describe an IV that has accessed surrounding tissues rather than the inside of the vein. This is also termed a "blown" IV line. (ECTSI 5, p. 789)

35: **B.** Because a butterfly is a plain steel needle, care must be taken to avoid moving it from side to side once it is within the confines of a vein. Should this movement occur, the sharp end of the needle will most likely lacerate the vein, and "blow" the IV line. (ECTSI 5, p. 789)

36: **C.** Orthostatic hypotension occurs when someone quickly sits up, causing a drop in blood pressure. This condition does not occur as a result of circulatory overload. (ECTSI 5, p. 791)

37: **D.** Blood pulsating back into the administration tubing of an IV bag hanging from the ceiling of the ambulance is a sure sign that an artery has been cannulated. (ECTSI 5, p. 791)

Chapter 26

38: **B.** When an IV attempt fails, bleeding from the vein produces a hematoma. The size of the hematoma can be limited by applying direct pressure and raising the extremity above the level of the heart until the bleeding stops. (ECTSI 5, p. 791)

39: **C.** If an artery is cannulated during an attempt to start an IV line, the catheter or needle must be removed immediately, and direct pressure applied for a minimum of 10 minutes, or until bleeding stops. (ECTSI 5, p. 791)

40: **A.** Thrombophlebitis is a late complication of IV therapy, but it is rarely seen in the prehospital setting. However, if you are called upon for a facility-to-facility transfer for a patient with a previously established IV, it could be noted. (ECTSI 5, p. 791)

41: **A.** Congestive heart failure is a condition characterized by the heart's inability to effectively circulate blood from the right side through the pulmonary system and out through the left ventricle. Initiating a large-bore IV line at a wide-open rate to such a patient's already impaired circulatory system will result in fluid overload and ultimately only worsen his or her condition. (ECTSI 5, p. 791)

42: **C.** An anaphylactic reaction can occur for a number of reasons: the IV fluid is contaminated; it has passed its expiration date; or the patient is allergic to the medication administered through the IV line. Of those listed, an allergy to the medication is the most common cause of an anaphylactic reaction. (ECTSI 5, p. 791)

43. **C.** Given the clinical signs in this situation, redness and swelling around the IV site, and a localized temperature increase, the patient most likely has an infection. The most appropriate course of action in this situation is to change the IV line to the other extremity. (ECTSI 5, p. 791)

44: **A.** IV fluids leaking into surrounding tissue will irritate the tissue, and the patient will often describe a burning sensation at the IV site. (ECTSI 5, p. 791)

45: **C.** When blood or blood products are introduced into the vascular system, it is called a transfusion. (ECTSI 5, p. 784)

46: **B.** Initiating IV therapy is not within the scope of performance of an EMT-A. Performing this therapy requires additional training as it is an invasive procedure. (ECTSI 5, p. 783)

47: **A.** When fluids such as colloids or crystalloids are introduced into the vasculature, it is called an infusion. (ECTSI 5, p. 784)

Intravenous Therapy

48: **C.** Hanging the IV bag too high above the patient would only help it to flow faster, rather than slow or stop it. (ECTSI 5, p. 790)

49: **C.** Infusion of cold IV fluid into a patient, especially if a large amount of fluid is infused quickly, can result in hypothermia. (ECTSI 5, p. 791)

50: **D.** Fainting, air embolism, and circulatory overload are all systemic complications of IV therapy. Tissue sloughing is a local complication. (ECTSI 5, p. 791)

Chapter 27

Advanced Airway Management

Chapter Goals

The exercises in this chapter are designed to help the student to:

- list the equipment needed to perform advanced airway management techniques.

- describe the steps in performing intubation with an endotracheal tube.

- describe the steps in performing intubation with an esophageal obturator airway.

- identify circumstances in which different advanced airway management techniques should be used.

- describe complications of advanced airway management.

Advanced Airway Management

Multiple-Choice Questions

Select the correct answer for each of the following questions. Each question has only *one* correct or best answer.

1. Which of the following would be considered a lethal complication of endotracheal intubation?

    A. Accidentally chipping the patient's two front teeth

    B. Ventilating without giving the patient supplemental oxygen

    C. Intubating the esophagus, and not recognizing it

    D. Hyperextending the cervical spine of a nontrauma patient

2. The principal reason for hyperventilating a patient before attempting intubation is to:

    A. increase carbon dioxide levels.

    B. increase oxygen saturation.

    C. constrict the patient's pupils.

    D. decrease hydrogen ion concentration.

3. Your first attempt to intubate a patient takes 30 seconds and is unsuccessful. Your next step should be to:

    A. perform a surgical cricothyrotomy.

    B. suction the patient for 15 to 20 seconds.

    C. immediately attempt to intubate the patient again.

    D. ventilate the patient with high-flow oxygen for 2 to 3 minutes.

Chapter 27

4. You insert an ET tube in an unconscious 48-year-old patient who has a head injury. You then begin to hyperventilate the patient with a bag-valve-mask device attached to an oxygen reservoir at a rate of 24 breaths per mintue. The principal goal of hyperventilation is to:

   A. prevent pneumothorax.

   B. decrease oxygen saturation.

   C. decrease intracranial pressure.

   D. increase retention of carbon dioxide.

5. After intubating a patient, you should auscultate all of the following areas **EXCEPT** the:

   A. right lung.

   B. left lung.

   C. area over the epigastrium.

   D. area above the suprasternal notch.

6. Immediately after inserting an endotracheal tube, you notice that the patient has no breath sounds on the left side. You suspect that you have inadvertently:

   A. intubated the right main stem bronchus.

   B. intubated the left main stem bronchus.

   C. placed the ET tube in the carina.

   D. placed the ET tube into the pyriform sinus.

7. The most important step in airway management of a patient who has a flail chest segment in the left axillary area is to:

   A. tape the flail segment into place.

   B. transport the patient lying on the unaffected side.

   C. administer oxygen at 2 L/min via nasal cannula.

   D. provide vigorous respiratory support with high-flow oxygen.

Advanced Airway Management

8. Laryngospasm might occur if a laryngoscope is inserted into the posterior pharynx of a child who has:

   A. croup.

   B. epiglottitis.

   C. pneumonia.

   D. bronchiolitis.

9. A patient who has taken an overdose of a narcotic may require intubation and assisted ventilations due to:

   A. increasing intracranial pressure.

   B. severe respiratory depression.

   C. moderate hypertension.

   D. the absence of a gag reflex.

10. Which of the following is considered a common side effect of nasopharyngeal intubation?

    A. Epistaxis

    B. Headaches

    C. Hypotension

    D. Chipped teeth

11. Tracheal deviation, distended neck veins, progressive hypotension, and a bulging chest may suggest that a patient has a:

    A. flail chest.

    B. hemothorax.

    C. ruptured esophagus.

    D. tension pneumothorax.

Chapter 27

12. Which of the following actions is **NOT** proper technique for suctioning?

    A. Suctioning for 20 to 30 seconds

    B. Lubricating the tip of the catheter

    C. Applying suction when withdrawing the catheter

    D. Administering oxygen before and after suctioning

13. Auscultation of breath sounds is an important aspect of all of the following procedures **EXCEPT**:

    A. before the application of a PASG.

    B. before performing a venipuncture.

    C. after placement of an ET tube.

    D. after placement of an esophageal Combitube.

14. Which of the following conditions is **NOT** considered a side effect of extended suctioning?

    A. Hypoxia

    B. Hypoxemia

    C. Cardiac irritability

    D. Gastric distention

15. Which of the following is a contraindication for using the esophageal obturator airway (EOA)?

    A. Cardiac arrest

    B. Pediatric patient

    C. Heroin overdose

    D. Respiratory arrest

Advanced Airway Management

16. The cuff on the ET tube that is used to seal the trachea can normally be inflated with how many milliliters of air?

    A. 5 to 10

    B. 20 to 30

    C. 30 to 50

    D. 50 to 75

17. Which of the following is **NOT** considered an advantage of endotracheal intubation?

    A. It prevents aspiration.

    B. It promotes gastric distention.

    C. It facilitates airway suctioning.

    D. It facilitates oxygen administration.

18. Most adult males will need approximately what size ET tube?

    A. 3.0 to 4.0 mm

    B. 5.5 to 6.5 mm

    C. 7.5 to 8.0 mm

    D. 9.5 to 10.0 mm

19. The plastic-coated wire inserted into an ET tube that makes the tube rigid, yet maintains a desired curvature, is called a:

    A. J-wire.

    B. stylet.

    C. French catheter.

    D. double lumen wire.

Chapter 27

20. The laryngoscope blade is used primarily to:

    A. lift the ET tube into the proper place.

    B. prevent the patient from vomiting.

    C. provide a direct view of the vocal cords.

    D. lift the uvula out of the field of vision.

21. When an ET tube is properly positioned, the upper edge of the balloon should lie approximately:

    A. 1" below the vocal cords.

    B. 1 1/2" above the vocal cords.

    C. 2" below the vocal cords.

    D. 2 1/2" above the vocal cords.

22. What type of special forceps is used to grasp objects obstructing the airway?

    A. Macintosh

    B. Miller

    C. Magill

    D. Mumbo

23. Insertion of an ET tube should take about how long?

    A. No more than 10 seconds

    B. 30 seconds or less

    C. 45 to 60 seconds

    D. 1 to 2 minutes

24. When attempting oral intubation on a trauma patient, it is important to:

    A. use one size larger ET tube than normal.

    B. maintain manual spinal immobilization.

    C. inflate the cuff with an extra 15 mL of air.

    D. avoid using a stylet to facilitate placement.

Advanced Airway Management

25. An end tidal CO_2 detector is used primarily to:

    A. assist in confirming the proper placement of an ET tube.

    B. measure and monitor a patient's carbon monoxide level.

    C. evaluate a patient's neurologic status after performing CPR.

    D. warn rescuers that they are entering a hazardous environment.

26. One advantage to using an esophageal obturator airway (EOA) is that it:

    A. does not require visualization of the vocal cords for placement.

    B. works well on patients who have ingested caustic substances.

    C. can be safely used on children who are less that 48" tall.

    D. has no adverse effects if it is placed in the trachea.

27. The esophageal obturator airway (EOA) is designed to be placed with the patient's head in what position?

    I. Slightly flexed
    II. Hyperextended
    III. Neutral

    A. I only

    B. I and III only

    C. II and III only

    D. I. II, and III

28. The PtL airway is designed to provide lung ventilation when it is placed in the:

    A. trachea.

    B. esophagus.

    C. trachea or esophagus.

    D. none of the above.

Chapter 27

29. One of the problems associated with advanced airway management is that:

    A. the risk of harming the patient is great.

    B. no specialized equipment is required.

    C. the skills are easily performed without special training.

    D. medical control and quality assurance are unimportant.

30. Which of the following is considered the "gold standard" or definitive method of securing an airway?

    A. Bag-valve-mask device

    B. Endotracheal intubation

    C. Esophageal obturator airway

    D. Esophageal gastric tube airway

31. You have just placed an esophageal obturator airway (EOA) when the patient regains consciousness. The most appropriate course of action would be to first position the patient properly and then:

    A. leave the airway in place until the patient is seen by a physician.

    B. replace the airway with an EGTA immediately.

    C. remove the airway, but be alert for vomiting.

    D. perform a needle cricothyrotomy.

32. Improper positioning of the EOA/EGTA can be confirmed by:

    A. absence of breath sounds on one or both sides.

    B. midline and reactive pupils.

    C. the presence of equal breath sounds in all fields.

    D. the patient regaining consciousness spontaneously.

Advanced Airway Management

33. Which of the following statements about the EOA is **FALSE**?

    A. It requires extreme force to place correctly.

    B. It blocks the esophagus and prevents aspiration.

    C. It cannot be used on children.

    D. It cannot be used on patients with esophageal disease.

34. What is the most common complication associated with the use of an EOA/EGTA?

    A. Hypocarbia

    B. Accidental placement in the trachea

    C. Inability to inflate the cuff

    D. Pronounced gastric distention

35. You insert an EOA properly, but the patient continues to show signs of inadequate ventilation. The most likely reason for continued breathing difficulty is:

    A. persistent leakage of air around the face mask.

    B. a ruptured balloon on the end of the EOA.

    C. presence of a tension pneumothorax.

    D. placement of the EOA in the trachea.

36. Which of the following statements about the PtL airway is **FALSE**?

    A. A mask seal is not necessary.

    B. It is easy to use in patients with spinal injuries.

    C. The device still works, even if the cuff malfunctions.

    D. It protects the airway from upper airway secretions.

Chapter 27

37. At what anatomical point does the trachea divide into the right and left main stem bronchi?

    A. Carina

    B. Septum

    C. Angle of Louis

    D. Suprasternal notch

38. The curved laryngoscope blade is designed to be placed into the:

    A. vallecula.

    B. carina.

    C. uvula.

    D. nares.

39. Which of the following statements about demand valve resuscitators is **FALSE**?

    A. It is possible to deliver 100% oxygen to the patient.

    B. Prolonged use often produces gastric distention.

    C. They provide flow rates of 40 to 50 L/min.

    D. They work well on infants and children.

40. The Venturi mask has a special design that makes it particularly useful for use with what type of patients?

    A. Trauma patients

    B. Pediatric patients

    C. COPD patients

    D. Overdose patients

Advanced Airway Management

Answers

1: **C.** While all of the options represent complications of endotracheal intubation, the only lethal complication is the unrecognized and uncorrected placement of an ET tube into the esophagus. (ECTSI 5, p. 796)

2: **B.** Before attempting intubation, a patient must be well oxygenated. A patient who is not hyperventilated with 100% oxygen before intubation may quickly desaturate during the process. (ECTSI 5, p. 798)

3: **D.** In most cases, patients undergoing endotracheal intubation are not breathing. As a result, they will desaturate during the intubation process as oxygen levels drop and carbon dioxide levels rise. Therefore, patients should be hyperventilated for 2 to 3 minutes prior to a second attempt at intubation. This is true even in patients who have been hyperventilated prior to a first attempt at intubation, but to a much lesser extent. If after two attempts, the tube cannot be passed, another ventilation technique should be used or another qualified rescuer should attempt to intubate. (ECTSI 5, p. 803)

4: **C.** Decreasing carbon dioxide levels through controlled hyperventilation at a rate of approximately 20 to 30 breaths a minute produces vasoconstriction, which in turn helps reduce intracranial pressure. (ECTSI 5, pp. 328–329, 798)

5: **D.** Auscultating over both lungs and over the epigastrium helps to confirm that the tube is properly placed in the trachea rather than in the esophagus. (ECTSI 5, p. 800)

6: **A.** Pushing the ET tube in too far past the vocal cords will cause it to enter the right main stem bronchus, which in turn will only allow ventilation of the right lung. (ECTSI 5, p. 801)

7: **D.** Flail chest often results in breathing difficulties first because the pain of the fractured ribs causes the patient to breath fast and shallow. In addition, flail chest is commonly associated with pulmonary contusion. Vigorous respiratory support, such as positive pressure ventilation, with high-flow oxygen, (and occasionally in conjunction with intubation) is required, along with rapid transport to the emergency department. (ECTSI 5, p. 378)

Chapter 27

8: **B.** Simply touching the inflamed, swollen epiglottis of a child with epiglottitis can result in total occlusion of the airway, which can then only be restored with a surgical airway. As such, direct laryngoscopy of a patient believed to have epiglottitis would be contraindicated. (ECTSI 5, p. 562)

9: **B.** A narcotic overdose will produce respiratory depression. As a result respirations will be both infrequent and shallow. (ECTSI 5, p. 528)

10: **A.** Slight bleeding may occur even when a nasopharyngeal airway is inserted properly. Therefore, whenever you attempt to insert a nasopharyngeal airway, remember to lubricate the tube prior to insertion. It is also important to select an airway device that is small enough to pass without having to force it. (ECTSI 5, p. 172)

11: **D.** These are the classic signs of a tension pneumothorax, which may develop as a traumatic chest injury progresses. This is a life-threatening condition in which prehospital care includes either release of an occlusive dressing if it occurs following the bandaging of an open chest wound, or needle decompression by appropriately trained ALS personnel. (ECTSI 5, p. 381)

12: **A.** Suctioning for prolonged periods of time will leave the patient severely hypoxic and can have serious side effects. (ECTSI 5, p. 176)

13: **B.** Auscultation of breath sounds would be important in all of the procedures listed, except for the venipuncture, where it would have no use. (ECTSI 5, pp. 215–216, 795)

14: **D.** All of the conditions listed, except gastric distention, could result from extended suctioning. (ECTSI 5, p. 176)

15: **B.** Due to the length of the EOA tube, its use is contraindicated in patients younger than 16 years. (ECTSI 5, p. 807)

16: **A.** If the proper size ET tube has been selected, it should take no more than 5 to 10 mL of air to inflate the cuff and secure the airway. Overinflation may result in a blown cuff, or in damage to the patient's trachea or vocal cords. (ECTSI 5, p. 800)

17: **B.** Endotracheal intubation will prevent gastric distention rather than promote it, as intubation isolates the airway from the stomach. (ECTSI 5, p. 796)

Advanced Airway Management

18: **C.** Most adult males will need a 7.5- or 8-mm diameter ET tube. (ECTSI 5, p. 796)

19: **B.** The plastic-coated wire inserted into an ET tube that makes the tube rigid, yet able to maintain a desired curvature, is called a stylet. (ECTSI 5, p. 797)

20: **C.** The laryngoscope blade is used primarily to lift the epiglottis out of the way to provide a direct view of the vocal cords. A straight blade will physically lift the epiglottis. A curved blade is inserted into the vallecula and causes the epiglottis to lift because of its anatomical connection. (ECTSI 5, p. 799)

21: **A.** When an ET tube is properly positioned, the upper edge of the balloon should lie approximately 1" below the level of the vocal cords. At this depth, the cuff on the ET tube will function best to secure the airway, and there is less likelihood that the tube will enter the right main stem bronchus. (ECTSI 5, p. 800)

22: **C.** Magill forceps are special forceps that can be used to grasp objects obstructing the airway. (ECTSI 5, p. 798)

23: **B.** Lengthy attempts at intubating (longer than 30 seconds) can result in severe hypoxia, especially if the patient is not adequately hyperventilated with high-flow oxygen before the attempt at intubation. (ECTSI 5, p. 801)

24: **B.** Maintaining an open airway is the top priority for all patients. When the airway of a trauma patient cannot be secured with less invasive methods, inserting an ET tube will be necessary. However, if you must intubate the patient, your partner should kneel straddling the patient and provide manual spinal immobilization to limit movement of the cervical spine during intubation. (ECTSI 5, p. 802)

25: **A.** One use of an end tidal CO_2 detector is to confirm proper placement of an ET tube, as the detector reacts to levels of carbon dioxide produced during exhalation. (ECTSI 5, p. 803)

26: **A.** One advantage to using an EOA is that a laryngoscope is not needed to visualize the vocal cords during intubation. (ECTSI 5, p. 804)

27: **B.** The esophageal obturator airway (EOA) is designed to be placed with the patient's head in a slightly flexed (or neutral with a trauma patient) position. Placing the head in this position helps to increase the likelihood that the tube will enter the esophagus rather than the trachea. (ECTSI 5, p. 805)

Chapter 27

28: **C.** The unique dual lumen design of the PtL airway allows it to function whether it is placed in the trachea or the esophagus. (ECTSI 5, p. 809)

29: **A.** With all advanced airway techniques comes increased risk to the patient due to the fact that these procedures are invasive. As such, it is always important to assess the risks and benefits to the patient when considering performing these techniques. (ECTSI 5, p. 812)

30: **B.** Endotracheal intubation is considered the definitive airway in prehospital as well as in-hospital patient care. (ECTSI 5, p. 796)

31: **C.** Due to its anatomical location when properly placed, the EOA can stimulate vomiting when it is removed. Therefore, it is best to be alert and have suctioning equipment available prior to removing the EOA. (ECTSI 5, p. 807)

32: **A.** The absence of breath sounds on one or both sides of the chest indicates that the EOA/EGTA has been inserted into the trachea or the right main stem bronchus. If this is the case, the airway should be removed and reinserted. (ECTSI 5, p. 808)

33: **A.** Proper technique when placing the EOA requires virtually no force, much less extreme force. (ECTSI 5, p. 806)

34: **B.** The most common complication associated with the use of an EOA/EGTA is accidental placement into the trachea rather than the esophagus. If the patient is not properly positioned prior to attempting to place an EOA, the tube will most likely enter the trachea. (ECTSI 5, p. 808)

35: **A.** A patient will not be adequately ventilated without a tight seal around the face mask on the EOA. A firm seal of the mask against the face must be maintained at all times during the use of the EOA/EGTA. (ECTSI 5, p. 808)

36: **C.** Occasionally the cuff on the PtL airway will leak. Cuff malfunction will result in improper functioning, and the patient's airway will not be protected. (ECTSI 5, pp. 811–812)

37: **A.** The trachea ends at the carina by dividing into smaller tubes, the right and left main stem bronchi. (ECTSI 5, p. 103)

38: **A.** The curved blade is designed to be inserted into the vallecula, after which a lifting motion will cause the epiglottis to lift up and out of the way, allowing an unobstructed view of the vocal cords. (ECTSI 5, p. 799)

Advanced Airway Management

39: **D.** Demand valve resuscitators are not designed to be used on infants or children. (ECTSI 5, p. 185)

40. **C.** The Venturi mask is commonly used on patients who have chronic obstructive pulmonary disease (COPD). The unique design features of the Venturi mask allow it to deliver specific concentrations of oxygen, which is important if patients with COPD are receiving extended oxygen therapy. (ECTSI 5, p. 183)

Chapter 28

Defibrillation for EMTs

Chapter Goals

The exercises in this chapter are designed to help the student to:

- identify parts of the electrical system of the heart.

- recognize basic arrhythmias.

- describe the defibrillation equipment and its maintenance.

- explain the steps of defibrillation.

- identify problems that may occur during defibrillation.

Defibrillation for EMTs

Multiple-Choice Questions

Select the correct answer for each of the following questions. Each question has only *one* correct or best answer.

1. Cardiac monitoring of a patient in cardiac arrest shows ventricular fibrillation. Of the following, which step is the most important in providing lifesaving patient care?

    A. Cardiopulmonary resuscitation

    B. Rapid defibrillation

    C. Oxygen administration

    D. Transport to the cardiac care unit

2. Interference in ECG signals is correctly referred to as:

    A. asystole.

    B. artifact.

    C. cardiac standstill.

    D. the isoelectric line.

3. Which of the following is a portable, battery-powered device used to record cardiac rhythm and to deliver electrical shocks?

    A. Monitor/defibrillator

    B. Pulse oxymeter

    C. Heart/lung resuscitator

    D. Transvenous pacemaker

4. The coordinated pumping contractions of a healthy heart produce which of the following cardiac rhythms?

    A. Ventricular tachycardia

    B. Normal sinus rhythm

    C. Pulseless electrical activity

    D. Torsade de pointes

Chapter 28

5. A cardiac rhythm that shows a flat line with a weak QRS complex of less than once every 5 to 10 seconds would be correctly identified as:

   A. an artifact.

   B. an agonal rhythm.

   C. a sinus rhythm with PVCs.

   D. a run of ventricular tachycardia.

6. The electrical charge generated and delivered by a defibrillator is called:

   A. pulsus paradoxus.

   B. a pacemaker spike.

   C. a QRS complex.

   D. a countershock.

7. Which of the following are considered lethal arrhythmias that can be treated and terminated with a defibrillator?

   I. Ventricular fibrillation
   II. Asystole
   III. Pulseless ventricular tachycardia

   A. I only

   B. I and III only

   C. II and III only

   D. I, II, and III

8. Complete absence of heart activity is called:

   A. asystole.

   B. depolarization.

   C. pulseless electrical activity.

   D. premature ventricular contractions.

Defibrillation for EMTs

9. Which of the following is **NOT** a skill required for a manual EMT-D ?

    A. Initiating IV therapy

    B. Charging the defibrillator

    C. Recognizing ventricular fibrillation

    D. Delivering an electrical countershock

10. What is the leading cause of death in the United States?

    A. Cancer

    B. Trauma

    C. Overdose/poisoning

    D. Heart-related disease

11. Which of following factors is **NOT** associated with successful resuscitation of a patient in cardiac arrest?

    A. The collapse is observed by a witness who then begins CPR.

    B. The patient's ECG rhythm is ventricular fibrillation.

    C. EMS system responds within 4 to 6 minutes of the cardiac arrest.

    D. Defibrillation occurs within 12 to 14 minutes of the cardiac arrest.

12. Approximately how many people die suddenly of cardiac arrest each year in the United States?

    A. 50,000

    B. 125,000

    C. 350,000

    D. 750,000

Chapter 28

13. What is the one major difference between manual and automated defibrillators?

    A. Automated defibrillators need their batteries recharged, but manual defibrillators do not.

    B. Manual defibrillators shock patients at levels up to five times as high as automatic defibrillators.

    C. Automated defibrillators cannot recognize and identify ventricular tachycardia, but manual defibrillators can.

    D. Manual defibrillators require that the operator recognize shockable rhythms before delivering a shock to the patient.

14. What is the primary pacemaker in a normal, healthy heart?

    A. SA node

    B. A-V junction

    C. Bundle of His

    D. Purkinje fibers

15. Which of the following will **NOT** result in improper or irregular heart beats?

    A. Lack of oxygen

    B. Interruption of the electrical system of the heart

    C. Injury or death of a portion of the heart muscle

    D. Immediate administration of high-flow oxygen

16. A patient with which of the following cardiac rhythms may have a palpable pulse?

    A. Asystole/agonal rhythm

    B. Ventricular tachycardia

    C. Ventricular fibrillation

    D. Pulseless electrical activity

Defibrillation for EMTs

17. If ventricular tachycardia is not treated quickly, it will often rapidly change into which of the following rhythms?

    A. Asystole

    B. Normal sinus rhythm

    C. Ventricular fibrillation

    D. Sinus rhythm with PVCs

18. Immediate depolarization of all cardiac muscle and its conducting tissues with an electrical countershock is called:

    A. diastole.

    B. defibrillation.

    C. myocardial infarction.

    D. cardiopulmonary resuscitation.

19. The flow of electrical current through a network of specialized tissue in the normal, healthy heart will produce:

    A. myocardial ischemia.

    B. spontaneous respirations.

    C. smooth, coordinated contractions.

    D. a corresponding drop in blood pressure.

20. Which of the following is considered a classic sign of ventricular fibrillation?

    A. Hypertension

    B. A rapid, thready pulse

    C. Absence of blood pressure

    D. Extreme, prolonged anxiety

Chapter 28

21. An electrocardiogram supplies graphic information about the:

    A. oxygen saturation of the blood.

    B. patient's blood pressure readings.

    C. strength and regularity of the pulse.

    D. electrical current flowing through the heart.

22. Each mechanical contraction of the heart is associated with what two electrical processes?

    A. Ischemia and infarction

    B. Repolarization and respirations

    C. Defibrillation and depolarization

    D. Depolarization and repolarization

23. The period from the beginning of the P wave to the beginning of the QRS complex is called the:

    A. PR interval.

    B. isoelectric line.

    C. diastolic period.

    D. pathologic period.

24. Each of the small boxes on an ECG tracing represents how many seconds?

    A. 0.04

    B. 0.1

    C. 0.4

    D. 1.0

25. Depolarization of the ventricles produces the:

    A. P wave.

    B. T wave.

    C. U wave.

    D. QRS complex.

Defibrillation for EMTs

26. Depolarization of the atria produces the:

    A. P wave.

    B. T wave.

    C. U wave.

    D. QRS complex.

27. The width of a normal QRS complex is how many seconds?

    A. 0.12 or less

    B. More than 0.5

    C. Exactly 1.2

    D. Exactly 1.5

28. The SA node is located:

    A. high in the right atria.

    B. low in the left ventricle.

    C. within the ventricular septum.

    D. between the atria and the ventricles.

29. The repolarization of the ventricles is represented on the electrocardiogram by the:

    A. P wave.

    B. T wave.

    C. QRS complex.

    D. isoelectric line.

30. Research and clinical experience have clearly shown that the treatment of choice for ventricular fibrillation is:

    A. rapid defibrillation.

    B. high-flow oxygen therapy.

    C. living wills and DNR orders.

    D. cardiopulmonary resuscitation.

Chapter 28

31. Which of the following features is **NOT** characteristic of ventricular fibrillation?

    A. No regular rhythm

    B. Narrow QRS complexes

    C. Varying height or amplitude

    D. Irregular shaped ECG pattern

32. When a patient is in ventricular tachycardia, the cardiac pacemaker is:

    A. absent.

    B. in the ventricles.

    C. in the SA node.

    D. in the AV junction.

33. What are the two types of ventricular fibrillation?

    A. Fine and irregular

    B. Irregular and regular

    C. Coarse and regular

    D. Coarse and fine

34. Portable defibrillators for prehospital use usually use what type of battery as a main power source?

    A. Nickel-cadmium

    B. Lithium

    C. Dilithium

    D. Lead acid

Defibrillation for EMTs

35. With a manual defibrillator, a patient's cardiac rhythm can be monitored:

    I. through standard cardiac monitor electrodes.

    II. automatically and then analyzed by the machine.

    III. through the two paddles of the defibrillator.

    A. I only

    B. I and III only

    C. II and III only

    D. I, II, and III

36. Evaluation of a cardiac rhythm with the "quick look" or hand-held defibrillator paddles is often difficult due to:

    A. artifacts from paddle movement.

    B. the extreme weight of the paddles.

    C. the short length of the connecting cables.

    D. the complex operational design of the paddles.

37. Electrical resistance between the patient's skin and the defibrillator paddles can be lowered by using:

    A. special gel or defibrillator pads.

    B. 4x4 or gauze bandages.

    C. multi-trauma dressings.

    D. alcohol-soaked pads.

38. Hand-held paddles should be pressed onto the patient's chest with at least how many pounds of force?

    A. 2

    B. 5

    C. 12

    D. 25

Chapter 28

39. The electrical current delivered by defibrillators is measured in:

    A. joules.

    B. amps.

    C. milliliters.

    D. ohms.

40. What are the three cycles or steps of defibrillation?

    A. Assessment, treatment, and CPR

    B. Treatment, CPR, and continuing education

    C. Response, assessment, and treatment

    D. Response, treatment, and continuing education

41. Once a patient has been shocked out of ventricular fibrillation into another rhythm, you should immediately check for:

    A. asystole.

    B. pulse.

    C. pupillary reaction.

    D. decreased level of consciousness.

42. Manual defibrillators can deliver countershocks measuring from:

    A. 1 to 10 joules.

    B. 10 to 360 joules.

    C. 100 to 600 joules.

    D. 500 to 2,000 joules.

43. Which of the following would **NOT** result in artifact from cable movement?

    A. Patient movement during transport

    B. Muscle tremors

    C. Cardiopulmonary resuscitation

    D. Rigor mortis

Defibrillation for EMTs

44. Which of the following can cause 60-cycle interference on an ECG tracing?

    A. Electric blanket

    B. Charcoal grill

    C. Dry, old electrodes

    D. Cardiopulmonary resuscitation

45. Which of the following will **NOT** result in artifact on an ECG tracing?

    A. Hairy chest

    B. Excessive sweating

    C. Dry electrodes

    D. Checking an apical pulse

46. What type of defibrillator batteries require regular charging and discharge cycles to maintain optimum performance?

    A. Lead acid

    B. Nickel cadmium

    C. Lithium

    D. Dilithium

47. What type of defibrillator batteries require no maintenance and have an extremely long shelf life?

    A. Lead acid

    B. Nickel cadmium

    C. Lithium

    D. Dilithium

Chapter 28

48. Which of the following interventions performed during defibrillation would **NOT** pose a risk to the rescuer or other rescuers?

    A. Starting an IV

    B. Intubating the patient

    C. Stopping CPR

    D. Moving the patient

49. The normal flow of electrical current through the heart monitored in lead II is from the:

    A. left shoulder to the left leg.

    B. left shoulder to the right leg.

    C. right shoulder to the left leg.

    D. right shoulder to the left shoulder.

50. During manual defibrillation of an adult patient, the defibrillator paddles are normally placed:

    A. on the right midaxillary line and the left midaxillary line.

    B. on the anterior chest, over the right and left nipples.

    C. at the upper right sternal border and the left midaxillary line.

    D. at the upper left sternal border and the right midaxillary line.

Answers

1: **B.** The single most important step in providing lifesaving care is rapid defibrillation. While the other steps are important in the overall care of the cardiac patient, rapid defibrillation is without question the single most important factor. The longer the patient remains in ventricular fibrillation, the harder it is to get him or her out of it.
(ECTSI 5, pp. 159–160)

2: **B.** Interference in ECG signals is correctly referred to as artifact.
(ECTSI 5, p. 823)

Defibrillation for EMTs

3: **A.** A monitor/defibrillator actually has two functions: it monitors cardiac rhythms and records those rhythms on paper; and it delivers either a random electrical countershock (defibrillation) or a synchronized shock (cardioversion). (ECTSI 5, p. 815)

4: **B.** The coordinated pumping contractions of the healthy, normal heart produce normal sinus rhythm. It implies that the SA node, the normal pacemaker of the heart, is in charge and functioning properly. (ECTSI 5, p. 819)

5: **B.** A cardiac rhythm that shows a flat line with a weak QRS complex of less than once every 5 to 10 seconds is representative of an agonal or dying heart rhythm. This rhythm may be seen just before asystole. (ECTSI 5, p. 820)

6: **D.** Defibrillation is a random countershock in the cardiac cycle; you push the buttons and the defibrillator delivers the charge. Cardioversion is a synchronized countershock; you push the buttons and the defibrillator looks for the top of a QRS complex, and then delivers the charge, avoiding the T wave (the vulnerable portion of the cardiac cycle). (ECTSI 5, pp. 815–816)

7: **B.** While the defibrillator can be used to terminate other cardiac arrhythmias, ventricular fibrillation and pulseless ventricular tachycardia are both lethal arrhythmias that can be treated with this therapy. (ECTSI 5, p. 815)

8: **A.** Asystole is the term used to describe a "flat line" on the cardiac monitor and represents total absence of cardiac activity. (ECTSI 5, p. 817)

9: **A.** Initiating IV therapy is not within the scope of practice of an EMT-D. It is an intermediate or advanced EMT skill. (ECTSI 5, p. 783)

10: **D.** Heart-related disease, including conditions such as myocardial infarction (heart attack) and congestive heart failure, is the leading cause of death in the United States. (ECTSI 5, p. 816)

11: **D.** Defibrillation should be performed within 8 minutes (and even sooner if possible) of collapse. (ECTSI 5, p. 816)

12: **C.** Approximately 350,000 people die suddenly of cardiac arrest each year, many of them outside the hospital. Many more die of heart-related problems. (ECTSI 5, p. 816)

Chapter 28

13: **D.** Manual defibrillators require the EMT-D to identify and treat shockable rhythms. Automatic and semiautomatic (automated) defibrillators recognize shockable cardiac rhythms and will not deliver a shock unless the patient has a shockable rhythm. (ECTSI 5, p. 816)

14: **A.** Located high in the right atrium, the SA node is the pacemaker for a normal, healthy heart. (ECTSI 5, p. 819)

15: **D.** Quick administration of high-flow oxygen will not result in an improper or irregular heart beat. Oxygen therapy may cause the heart beat to slow down if the heart is working hard and already ischemic. However, this is the desired result of oxygen therapy. (ECTSI 5, p. 817)

16: **B.** On occasion, a patient in ventricular tachycardia will have palpable pulses, but the other three rhythms listed will not. (ECTSI 5, p. 817)

17: **C.** If untreated, ventricular tachycardia will rapidly deteriorate into ventricular fibrillation. Ventricular tachycardia is a faster than normal cardiac rhythm, and as such, it increases myocardial work load, oxygen consumption, and irritability. (ECTSI 5, p. 817)

18: **B.** Immediate depolarization of the entire heart with an electrical countershock is called defibrillation. This therapy gives one of the normal pacemakers in the heart a chance to regain control and produce a perfusing rhythm. (ECTSI 5, p. 817)

19: **C.** When the electrical currents produced in the heart are conducted properly, the heart responds with smooth, coordinated contractions that move blood through the circulatory system. (ECTSI 5, p. 817)

20: **C.** With ventricular fibrillation, there is no effective pumping (filling or emptying) of the heart, hence no blood pressure. A patient in ventricular fibrillation will have no pulse. (ECTSI 5, p. 817)

21: **D.** The electrocardiogram (ECG) monitors the electrical current that flows through the heart. The ECG does not evaluate mechanical function of the heart, only the potential for it. (ECTSI 5, p. 819)

22: **D.** Each mechanical contraction of the heart is associated with depolarization and repolarization. Depolarization, a process in which the electrical charges on the surface of the muscle cell change from positive to negative, results in contractions. Repolarization, a process in which the heart returns to its resting state, results in refilling of the heart as it readies itself to accept another electrical impulse and contract again. (ECTSI 5, p. 819)

Defibrillation for EMTs

23: **A.** The period from the beginning of the P wave to the beginning of the QRS complex is the PR interval. This interval represents the time it takes for the SA node to initiate an impulse, traverse the atria, and reach the AV junction. (ECTSI 5, p. 819)

24: **A.** Each small box on the ECG tracing represents 0.04 seconds, with each group of five small boxes representing 0.2 seconds (one large box). In turn, each group of five large boxes represents 1.0 second. (ECTSI 5, p. 819)

25: **D.** Depolarization of the ventricles produces the QRS complex, which has the largest amplitude of the cardiac cycle, hence its size and prominence. (ECTSI 5, p. 819)

26: **A.** In a normal functioning heart, depolarization of the atria produces the P wave. (ECTSI 5, p. 819)

27: **A.** The width of a normal QRS complex is 0.12 seconds or less. Once the electrical impulse reaches the AV junction, it should take no more than 0.12 seconds for the impulse to traverse the bundle of His, the right and left bundle branches, and the Purkinje system, as the ventricles respond by contracting. (ECTSI 5, p. 819)

28: **A.** The SA node is located high in the right atria. (ECTSI 5, p. 819)

29: **B.** Repolarization of the ventricles is represented on the ECG by the T wave. (ECTSI 5, p. 819)

30: **A.** The treatment of choice for ventricular fibrillation is rapid defibrillation. (ECTSI 5, p. 817)

31: **B.** With ventricular fibrillation, the overall electrical pattern is irregularly shaped, chaotic, and lacks any regular repeating features. Therefore, there are no narrow QRS complexes associated with ventricular fibrillation, as there is no regular conduction of electricity, nor coordinated contractions associated with it. (ECTSI 5, p. 820)

32: **B.** With ventricular tachycardia, the ventricles are beating too fast to circulate blood effectively. (ECTSI 5, p. 815)

33: **D.** When a heart first fibrillates, it produces "coarse" ventricular fibrillation. As the cardiac muscle becomes more ischemic and grows more tired, the electrical amplitude becomes smaller, producing "fine" ventricular fibrillation. (ECTSI 5, p. 821)

Chapter 28

34: **A.** Portable defibrillators for prehospital use usually use a rechargeable nickel-cadmium battery for a main power source. (ECTSI 5, p. 821)

35: **B.** With a manual defibrillator, a patient's cardiac rhythm can be monitored through either standard cardiac monitor electrodes or through the paddles. The defibrillator paddles may be used to "quick look" the patient, but they will usually produce more artifact. (ECTSI 5, p. 823)

36: **A.** If the defibrillator paddles are not held very still, any motion will be represented on the cardiac monitor as artifact. (ECTSI 5, p. 823)

37: **A.** The use of alcohol or other flammable liquids during a defibrillation attempt is unacceptable, and application of a dry dressing or bandage would not reduce electrical resistance. (ECTSI 5, p. 823)

38: **D.** Using 25 lb of pressure on the defibrillator paddles ensures good contact with the patient and helps facilitate good "penetration" of the electrical current rather than merely surface flow, which would not depolarize the heart. (ECTSI 5, p. 823)

39: **A.** The terms joules or watt-seconds are generally interchangeable when being used to describe the amount of electricity being delivered by a defibrillator. (ECTSI 5, p. 823)

40: **A.** The patient is assessed, determined to be in ventricular fibrillation, and then treated (i.e., defibrillated). If there is no successful conversion of the cardiac rhythm after defibrillation, CPR is begun until the patient can be prepared to receive additional electrical therapy. CPR will maintain circulation until ALS personnel can begin drug therapy to improve the potential for the heart to return to a perfusing rhythm. (ECTSI 5, p. 825)

41: **B.** Once a patient has been shocked out of ventricular fibrillation, you should immediately assess for a pulse, blood pressure, or spontaneous respirations. (ECTSI 5, p. 825)

42: **B.** At present, manual defibrillators can deliver countershocks measuring from 10 to 360 joules. A countershock of less than 10 joules would be ineffective, and one of greater than 360 joules may harm the myocardium. (ECTSI 5, p. 823)

43: **D.** A patient in rigor mortis will not move at all; therefore, there would be no artifact. (ECTSI 5, p. 826)

44: **A.** Any device or electrical appliance using AC current in close proximity to the patient may produce 60-cycle interference. (ECTSI 5, pp. 826–827)

Defibrillation for EMTs

45: **D.** All of the options except D can produce poor electrode contact and in turn produce artifact on the cardiac monitor. (ECTSI 5, p. 826)

46: **B.** One of the characteristics of nickel-cadmium batteries is their need to be exercised regularly, that is, charged and discharged on a regular basis. (ECTSI 5, p. 828)

47: **C.** Lithium batteries require no maintenance, but are generally used as a backup power supply rather than as a primary source of power. (ECTSI 5, p. 828)

48: **C.** Any contact with a patient during defibrillation, either direct (CPR) or indirect (intubating) should be avoided due to the risk of conducting electricity. (ECTSI 5, p. 825)

49: **C.** Just as the electrical current in a normal heart runs from the SA node in the upper right atrium down through the heart, so lead II monitors it. (ECTSI 5, p. 819)

50: **C.** Placing the paddles at the upper right sternal border at the level of the angle of Louis, and on the left midaxillary line over the apex of the heart are currently thought to produce the best potential for delivering the countershock to the heart. (ECTSI 5, p. 825)

Chapter 29

Case Studies

Chapter Goals

The exercises in this chapter are designed to help the student to:

- follow a multiple-step clinical scenario.

- analyze patient information and then choose an appropriate series of actions.

- identify important factors, other than physical condition, that require the attention of the EMT when providing patient care.

Case Studies

Multiple-Choice Questions

This chapter is made up of several clinical situations, which are followed by a series of multiple-choice questions that refer to the situation. Like the other chapters, there is only *one* correct or best answer for each question. Each question is linked to the scenario, but the questions are not dependent on each other. That is, you need not know the answer to one question in the scenario to answer the next question.

Questions 1-3 refer to the information below.

You are called to the home of a man who tells you he had chest pains, but that they are now gone. He dismisses the pains as gas. The man's wife is obviously upset and anxious about her husband. She insists that you take him to the hospital, but he refuses to go.

1. In this situation, you must immediately ask yourself:

    A. "How far away is the nearest hospital?"

    B. "Is the patient's pain truly gone?"

    C. "Can the patient make a competent decision about treatment?"

    D. "Did the patient eat something that may have caused gas?"

2. You and your partner accept the patient's refusal and leave, but later that day you learn the patient's condition became worse and he died at home. Which of the following legal concepts will most likely be tested in this situation?

    A. Sovereign immunity

    B. Presumptive negligence

    C. Implied consent

    D. Abandonment

3. You and your partner are asked about the specific circumstances in which you left the scene. What type of consent should have been documented?

    A. Informed consent

    B. Implied consent

    C. Effective consent

    D. Statutory consent

Chapter 29

Questions 4-5 refer to the information below.

You are caring for a woman who has been injured in an automobile accident when a man approaches and says that he is a doctor.

4. In this situation, the doctor is acting as a volunteer at the scene of an emergency. In most states, his actions would be protected from liability according to:

    A. sovereign immunity laws.

    B. governmental immunity laws.

    C. Good Samaritan laws.

    D. implied consent laws.

5. The doctor at the scene tells you to follow a course of treatment that you do not think is appropriate. Your most appropriate course of action would be to:

    A. follow his instructions since he is a doctor and knows more than you do.

    B. thank the doctor for his offer to help and then follow your own course of treatment.

    C. ask law enforcement officials at the scene to arrest him for impersonating a doctor.

    D. contact medical control for instructions.

Questions 6-7 refer to the information below.

You are called to a restaurant where a woman who is at least 8 months pregnant is choking on a piece of meat. She is grasping her throat and coughing as she tries to breathe.

6. What information about the patient is most important in determining whether she has a complete airway obstruction or a partial airway obstruction?

    A. She is coughing.

    B. She is pregnant.

    C. She is choking on meat.

    D. She is grasping her throat.

Case Studies

7. The Heimlich maneuver would be ineffective in this situation because:

    A. the patient will go into premature labor.

    B. the pharynx will not be swollen enough.

    C. only back blows will help clear a partial airway obstruction.

    D. air flow created by the thrusts will go around the obstruction.

Questions 8-10 refer to the information below.

You are called to a construction site and find a construction worker buried to midchest in a trench. Other workers are trying to dig him out. The patient is cyanotic and has a pulse of 100/min and shallow respirations of 20/min. The foreman says that it will take at least 10 minutes to clear the dirt from around the patient's chest.

8. Your first step in caring for this patient is to:

    A. give the patient high-flow oxygen.

    B. contact medical control for instructions.

    C. make sure his airway is clear and stays clear.

    D. make sure the scene is safe for you and your partner.

9. Given the patient's vital signs, which of the following supplemental oxygen devices would be most appropriate at this time?

    A. Nasal cannula

    B. Simple face mask

    C. Venturi mask

    D. Nonrebreathing mask

10. Even though the patient is given supplemental oxygen, he becomes even more cyanotic. His respirations are now at 32/min and are very labored. Supplemental oxygen should now be given with a:

    A. 48% Venturi mask at 12 L/min.

    B. nonrebreathing mask with a reservoir.

    C. bag-valve-mask device with an oxygen reservoir.

    D. bag-valve-mask device via emergency tracheostomy.

Chapter 29

Questions 11-12 refer to the information below.

As you open the airway of an elderly man who is not breathing, you do not feel, hear, or see any air exchange. You deliver two quick breaths, mouth-to-mask. The patient's chest does not rise, and your breaths meet no resistance, but the patient's stomach inflates with each breath.

11. Your attempts at rescue breathing have not been effective most likely because the:

    A. rescue breaths are too fast, and the air is going into the esophagus.

    B. patient has had a laryngectomy, and the breaths are exiting via the stoma.

    C. patient has an open pneumothorax, and the breaths are exiting via the wound.

    D. seal around the mask is inadequate, and the air is leaking out around the patient's cheeks.

12. To ensure that rescue breathing becomes effective for this patient, you should first:

    A. check for a pulse before you start ventilations.

    B. make a better seal with the mask and begin ventilations again.

    C. discard the pocket mask and perform slower mouth-to-mouth ventilations.

    D. reposition the head and then begin again using slower mouth-to-mask ventilations.

Questions 13-14 refer to the information below.

You and a friend, who is also an EMT, see an elderly woman collapse at a shopping mall. You both rush to her side. The patient is unresponsive and does not seem to be breathing. You send a bystander to call 9-1-1.

13. Your first step in caring for the patient is to:

    A. check for a carotid pulse.

    B. check for signs of significant external bleeding.

    C. check for breathing with the look-listen-feel method.

    D. open the airway with the head-tilt/chin-lift maneuver.

Case Studies

14. If the patient is not breathing, you should next:

    A. check for a carotid pulse.

    B. check for a Medic-Alert bracelet.

    C. check for a foreign body obstruction in her mouth.

    D. provide two mouth-to-mouth or mouth-to-mask ventilations.

Questions 15-16 refer to the information below.

You are called to the scene of an accident in which a car with a lone driver has hit a utility pole. Witnesses say that the accident just happened. The driver is not breathing, has no carotid pulse, and has widely dilated pupils. The driver is also being held in an upright position by the steering wheel. An extrication team has been called.

15. The first step in caring for this patient is to:

    A. establish an open airway.

    B. pronounce the patient dead.

    C. begin cutting the car door with the jaws of life.

    D. apply direct pressure to control any external bleeding.

16. Given the mechanism of injury and the position in which you find the patient, you suspect the patient's primary injury to be:

    A. a closed head injury.

    B. an internal chest injury.

    C. fractures to the lower extremities.

    D. myocardial infarction, which resulted in the accident.

Chapter 29

Questions 17-19 refer to the information below.

You are called to the home of a child who is injured in a bicycle accident. Upon arrival, you find the child sitting on the porch of his house, about 25' from the accident site. He tells you he skidded on some sand and then fell off the bicycle. He remembers everything that happened and that he only hurt his knee. You note an abrasion on the knee with a small amount of bleeding.

17. Given the circumstances in this situation, your first concern when assessing the patient is to:

    A. treat the knee injury.

    B. check for responsiveness.

    C. rule out any life-threatening problems.

    D. find and treat all injuries in the order you find them.

18. As you begin assessing the patient's knee, it would be most helpful to know:

    A. the child's age.

    B. the approximate speed of the bicycle.

    C. how the child got to the porch.

    D. how far the bicycle skidded before it stopped.

19. You decide to dress and bandage the abrasion and then splint the injured leg. Which of the following steps should be performed both before and after this intervention?

    A. Obtaining and recording a complete set of vital signs

    B. Obtaining consent from the patient's parents or guardians

    C. Consulting by radio or telephone with medical control

    D. Assessing distal motor function, sensation, and circulation in the injured leg

Case Studies

Questions 20-21 refer to the information below.

A 45-year-old man becomes caught in a machine at work, and his left arm is amputated between the wrist and the elbow. Upon your arrival, the patient has severe bleeding at the site, a blood pressure of 80/40 mm Hg, a weak pulse of 100/min, and shallow respirations of 24/min.

20. The patient's baseline vital signs suggest what type of shock?

    A. Psychogenic

    B. Neurogenic

    C. Hemorrhagic

    D. Metabolic

21. Your first attempt to control the bleeding should be with:

    A. a tourniquet.

    B. direct pressure.

    C. splinting and elevation.

    D. pressure on the arterial pressure points.

Questions 22-23 refer to the information below.

A woman has a closed depressed skull fracture after being thrown from her car when it crashed into a guard rail. The patient has a blood pressure of 160/110 mm Hg, a pulse of 50/min, and respirations of 24/min.

22. While the patient's combination of vital signs does not present a typical picture of shock, this pattern suggests:

    A. an allergic reaction.

    B. hypotensive crisis.

    C. increased intracranial pressure.

    D. the release of fat emboli from fractured bone ends.

Chapter 29

23. Your care for this patient should begin with providing proper spinal immobilization and:

    A. bandaging all open wounds.

    B. covering the patient with a blanket.

    C. giving supplemental oxygen.

    D. splinting the depressed skull fracture.

Questions 24-25 refer to the information below.

A 7-year-old girl fell out of the tree onto her right side. She cannot move her right arm, and she has a great deal of pain in the area of the right shoulder.

24. The principal goal in caring for the patient's extremity injury is to make sure to immobilize the involved bone or joint and:

    A. nothing else.

    B. the joints above and below the injury.

    C. the entire extremity below the injury.

    D. the entire extremity above the injury.

25. Given the mechanism of injury, the area of the greatest pain, and assuming there are no other serious injuries, which of the following devices should be used for immobilization?

    A. Traction splint

    B. Sling and swathe

    C. Cardboard splint following realignment

    D. The patient's uninjured arm for support in a position of comfort

Case Studies

Questions 26-28 refer to the information below.

A 15-year-old boy has pain in his right shoulder after being tackled in a football game. Upon arrival, you find the patient's football jersey and shoulder pads off, and the patient is holding the shoulder forward and lower than his uninjured shoulder. His vital signs are within normal limits. Gentle palpation of the injured area reveals deformity and pain between the shoulder and the neck.

26. Which of the following bones articulate to make up the shoulder girdle?

    A. Humerus, tibia, scapula

    B. Humerus, tibia, clavicle

    C. Scapula, clavicle, humerus

    D. Scapula, humerus, tibia

27. If the deformity between the patient's shoulder and neck is actually the head of the humerus, the patient's injury would be classified as:

    A. an open fracture.

    B. a closed fracture.

    C. an anterior dislocation.

    D. a posterior dislocation.

28. Appropriate immobilization of this patient would involve:

    A. bandaging the area.

    B. applying a traction splint.

    C. immobilizing the radius and ulna only.

    D. applying a sling and swathe over the entire extremity.

Chapter 29

Questions 29-31 refer to the information below.

An elderly woman falls on her hand after slipping on an icy sidewalk. You find her sitting in a nearby store, holding her right arm close to her chest. Her wrist appears to have a "silver fork" deformity.

29. Before you begin to immobilize the injury, you try to assess the motor function, sensation, and circulation in the injured hand. As you try to palpate the radial pulse, the patient cries out in pain. The most appropriate course of action would be to:

    A. assess the pulse in her thumb instead of in her wrist.

    B. assess capillary refill and skin condition instead of the pulse.

    C. advise medical control that you cannot assess her distal circulation.

    D. tell the patient that you must check her pulse, and then assess the pulse quickly.

30. As you prepare to splint the patient's injury, you should attempt to immobilize the injured arm:

    A. in the position of function.

    B. in a position of comfort.

    C. with adequate traction.

    D. against the side of the body.

31. Appropriate immobilization of this injury includes splinting which of the following bones?

    A. Radius and fibula

    B. Radius, humerus, and metacarpals

    C. Fibula and humerus

    D. Fibula and femur

Case Studies

Questions 32-33 refer to the information below.

A machine catches the hand of a 44-year-old factory worker resulting in a severe crush injury. The patient is holding his hand in a towel upon your arrival, but you note there is not much bleeding. However, the hand is obviously deformed, and the patient is in a great deal of pain. The patient has a blood pressure of 110/70 mm Hg, a pulse of 90/min, and respirations of 18/min. You estimate that transport will take at least 30 minutes due to developing blizzard conditions.

32. The patient's vital signs suggest:

    A. normal functioning.

    B. psychogenic shock.

    C. compensated shock.

    D. decompensated shock.

33. Of the following, which splint would be best for this injury?

    A. Air splint

    B. Pillow splint

    C. Traction splint

    D. Padded board splint

Questions 34-36 refer to the information below.

A man riding a motorcycle is struck from the side by an automobile. The patient is lying on the ground moaning upon your arrival. His face and lips are pale and ashen. There is marked deformity of the left thigh, but the skin is not broken. The patient has a blood pressure of 80/60 mm Hg, a weak pulse of 120/min, and respirations of 20/min.

34. The patient's vital signs suggest what type of shock?

    A. Anaphylactic shock

    B. Psychogenic shock

    C. Compensated shock

    D. Decompensated shock

Chapter 29

35. Based on the patient's vital signs and the mechanism of injury, the patient's shock is most likely due to:

    A. anaphylaxis.

    B. septicemia.

    C. internal bleeding.

    D. external bleeding.

36. The patient's physical findings suggest that one possible major injury is a:

    A. depressed skull fracture.

    B. tension pneumothorax.

    C. fractured femur.

    D. ruptured aorta.

Questions 37-39 refer to the information below.

A 10-year-old girl fractures her left femur as a result of falling from a skateboard. The bone ends are protruding through the skin, and there is visible bleeding. The patient has a blood pressure of 60/30 mm Hg, a thready pulse of 120/min, and shallow respirations of 30/min.

37. Your first step in caring for the patient's fracture is to apply:

    A. traction.

    B. a splint.

    C. manual pressure to realign the bone ends.

    D. manual pressure to control the bleeding.

38. As you and your partner prepare to apply a Hare Traction Splint to the patient's fractured femur, it is important to remember that the:

    A. ischial pad must be set firmly against the ilium.

    B. splint must extend 5 inches beyond the injured extremity.

    C. splint must be exactly the same length as the injured extremity.

    D. traction must be maintained as the ankle hitch is connected to the end of the splint.

348 Student Review Manual

Case Studies

39. One way to prevent the loss of traction when applying the traction splint is to:

    A. remove the ischial strap.

    B. attach the "cradles" before applying traction.

    C. place the ankle hitch around the ankle and foot before applying traction.

    D. make sure both you and your partner are applying traction at all times.

Questions 40-42 refer to the information below.

A man involved in an automobile accident is standing motionless next to his car upon your arrival. There is a "starburst" pattern on the windshield. The patient says that as he was explaining the accident to a police officer his neck began to hurt and his hands and feet began to "feel tingly." The patient's vital signs are within normal limits.

40. Given the patient's statements and the mechanism of injury, you should prepare to care for:

    A. an allergic reaction.

    B. an emotional crisis.

    C. a severed spinal cord.

    D. swelling or pressure on the spinal cord.

41. The fact that the patient is standing indicates that:

    A. spinal immobilization is not needed.

    B. the spinal cord and spinal column are safe.

    C. the spinal cord is safe.

    D. the spinal cord has not been severed yet.

Chapter 29

42. The proper way to prepare the patient for transport would be to:

    A. carry the stretcher to the patient and then ask him to sit down.

    B. ask him to walk to the ambulance and then sit down on the stretcher in the back.

    C. secure the patient to a short spine board and then lower him onto the stretcher.

    D. fully immobilize the patient on a long spine board while he is still standing and then lower the board onto the stretcher.

Questions 43-45 refer to the information below.

A four-member EMT team, in which you are the leader, is called to the scene of a two-car accident where 6 people are injured. Law enforcement, fire, and rescue teams are at the scene and at work.

43. You and your team are responsible for which of the following functions at this incident?

    A. Traffic control and patient care

    B. Fire suppression and patient care

    C. Vehicle rescue and patient care

    D. Patient care only

44. As leader of the EMT team, your first responsibility upon arrival at the scene should be to:

    A. begin triage immediately.

    B. begin providing patient care.

    C. assign patients to the team.

    D. coordinate with the incident commander.

45. Given the situation and the number of patients, you should next:

    A. call for more ambulances.

    B. quickly assess patients in the order you find them.

    C. assign one EMT for every two patients.

    D. assign one EMT to each car, with the other EMT assigned to help as needed.

Case Studies

Questions 46-48 refer to the information below.

A 19-year-old man who was stabbed in the upper right side of the chest is cyanotic and having difficulty breathing. The knife was removed by the patient's girlfriend before your arrival. The wound is "sucking air" and has been covered with an occlusive bandage by a first responder. En route to the hospital, the patient's cyanosis deepens, he has even more difficulty breathing, and his pulse and blood pressure indicate increasing shock. You notice that the patient's trachea has moved from the midline to the uninjured side.

46. The mechanism of injury and the patient's current signs and symptoms suggest:

    A. cardiac tamponade.

    B. a pneumothorax.

    C. a hemopneumothorax.

    D. a tension pneumothorax.

47. The principal difference between pneumothorax and hemothorax is that with pneumothorax:

    A. blood pools in the pleural space.

    B. blood oozes into the tissues around the lungs.

    C. small bubbles of air leak from the lungs and come to lie in the subcutaneous tissue.

    D. air leaks into the pleural space from an opening in the chest or the lung.

48. Immediate treatment of the patient's deteriorating condition should include:

    A. giving the patient oxygen and waiting for an ALS unit to arrive.

    B. performing mouth-to-mask ventilations to reinflate the lungs.

    C. releasing one corner of the occlusive dressing to release the accumulated air.

    D. releasing one corner of the occlusive dressing to allow the accumulated blood to drain.

Chapter 29

Questions 49-52 refer to the information below.

A small car with two passengers crashes into a utility pole, resulting in two power lines falling over the car. A man is lying on the ground approximately 20' from the car. A woman is lying partially out of the car with one leg on the ground. Your partner begins assessing the man.

49. Your first step is to:

    A. open the woman's airway.

    B. attach the cardiac monitor to the woman's chest.

    C. call the utility company to shut off the power.

    D. assess the woman's level of consciousness.

50. Your partner finds the man pulseless and unresponsive. He applies the "quick look" paddles and sees a total absence of electrical activity on the cardiac monitor. The cardiac rhythm consistent with this description is called:

    A. asystole.

    B. junctional rhythm.

    C. normal sinus rhythm.

    D. ventricular fibrillation.

51. The fire department has now removed the woman from the car. You begin cardiac monitoring and confirm that the patient is in fine ventricular fibrillation. You should immediately:

    A. begin CPR.

    B. start an IV line.

    C. defibrillate the patient.

    D. give high-flow oxygen.

Case Studies

52. You begin to provide patient care without making radio contact, based on written directions from your medical director. You are following:

    A. standing orders.

    B. an advance directive.

    C. the law of informed consent.

    D. directives from a living will.

Questions 53-56 refer to the information below.

You are called to a construction site where a first responder meets you and states that a teenager is buried in a large pile of sand. The patient was playing with friends on a large sandpile when the sand began to shift and buried him completely except for his right hand. His friends tried to pull him out, but were unable to do so as the sand kept shifting. The patient has been submerged for about 5 or 6 minutes. The patient has a weak pulse, but as you pull him from the sand, find that he is having difficulty breathing. His face is flushed and purple, his neck veins are distended, and his eyes are bulging and bloodshot.

53. Your first step is to:

    A. begin CPR.

    B. call for air medical support.

    C. open the airway.

    D. get the suction unit.

54. The patient's signs and symptoms suggest:

    A. traumatic asphyxia.

    B. neurogenic shock.

    C. massive hemothorax.

    D. hypovolemic shock.

Chapter 29

55. As you begin intubation, the patient starts to gag. Applying pressure over what anatomical structure will reduce the chance of vomiting into the upper airway?

    A. Suprasternal notch

    B. Carotid arteries

    C. Cricoid cartilage

    D. Nasal septum

56. After intubating the patient, you note an absence of breath sounds on the left side, most likely due to:

    A. inadequate tidal volume in the bag-valve-mask device.

    B. a faulty cuff on the endotracheal tube.

    C. inadequate oxygen flow to the bag-valve-mask device.

    D. intubation of the right main stem bronchus.

Questions 57-59 refer to the information below.

You are called to a local park where a family picnic is being held. Upon arrival, you see 6 people standing around an elderly man who is lying on the grass. As you approach the patient, he appears motionless and his skin appears blue. A young woman is holding the patient's hand and states, "Gramps just fell to the ground for no reason." She also states nothing has been done for the patient before your arrival and that the patient has been seeing a family doctor frequently for the past 6 months.

57. The first step in this situation would be to:

    A. ask a family member about the patient's medical history.

    B. get the names of all the eyewitnesses.

    C. ask what medications the patient is taking.

    D. make sure that the scene is safe.

Case Studies

58. Your partner moves to the patient's side. His first step in this situation would be to:

    A. give the patient two quick breaths.

    B. assess the patient's level of consciousness.

    C. begin CPR.

    D. give high-flow oxygen via nasal cannula.

59. Attempts to resuscitate the patient fail. Which of the following factors most likely contributed?

    A. The patient collapsed in front of several family members.

    B. No BLS measures were provided prior to your arrival.

    C. The patient is being treated outside at a park rather than at a hospital.

    D. No one is sure what medications he is taking.

Questions 60-62 refer to the information below.

You and your partner are called to a private family dwelling for an unknown emergency on a hot July day. As you pull into the driveway, you are met by a hysterical 10-year-old girl who just found her 2-year-old sister at the bottom of their swimming pool. The girl also tells you her mother "ran to the store for some milk." Once in the backyard, you see a small child lying on the bottom of a pool in 4' of water.

60. Your first step in this situation should be to:

    A. begin CPR.

    B. get permission to treat from the mother.

    C. apply a properly sized cervical collar.

    D. remove the child from the swimming pool.

61. What is the proper method for opening the patient's airway?

    A. Chin-lift technique

    B. Head-tilt/chin-lift technique

    C. Jaw-thrust technique

    D. Any technique will work.

Chapter 29

62. The patient has a weak pulse, but no respirations, suggesting:

    A. respiratory arrest.

    B. cardiac standstill.

    C. metabolic alkalosis.

    D. profound hypocarbia.

Questions 63-65 refer to the information below.

You are called to a local motel for a "man down." Upon your arrival, an employee points down the hall to where the patient's room is located. A small crowd has gathered outside the open door. You enter a small, filthy room littered with empty wine bottles to find a middle-aged man lying supine in bed. He has no pulse or respirations, and his skin is cool and dry. There is a marked purplish discoloration on his back and buttocks.

63. The discoloration on the back and buttocks is called:

    A. livor mortis.

    B. decomposition.

    C. acute pallor.

    D. putrefaction.

64. The most appropriate course of action in this situation would be to:

    A. start CPR immediately, unless a living will is present.

    B. contact medical control for instructions.

    C. request an ALS unit to the scene.

    D. refrain from starting CPR.

Case Studies

65. Which of the following factors are the most significant with regard to your decisions about providing patient care?

    A. Age of the patient and the empty wine bottles

    B. Cool, dry skin and the purplish discoloration

    C. Cool, dry skin and the empty wine bottles

    D. The position in which the patient was found and the filthy environment

Questions 66-70 refer to the information below.

Three golfers stand under a tree during a severe thunderstorm. Upon arrival, you find the three patients still under the tree. The first patient is a 40-year-old woman who appears confused, but is walking around. The second patient is a 42-year-old man who is obviously cyanotic and lying motionless on the ground. The third patient is a 75-year-old woman who is pale, but sitting up against the tree.

66. Which of the patients should be assessed first?

    A. The 40-year-old woman

    B. The 42-year-old man

    C. The 75-year-old woman

    D. The order does not matter.

67. Which of the following pulses would be most appropriate to assess in any of these patients?

    A. Radial

    B. Carotid

    C. Dorsalis pedis

    D. Posterior tibialis

Chapter 29

68. The 40-year-old woman states that the lightning strike occurred about 10 minutes ago, and that the man on the ground has been unresponsive and cyanotic since then. You suspect that the man will most likely:

    A. resuscitate very quickly if an ALS unit is called to the scene.

    B. regain consciousness on his own, if he is left alone.

    C. have minimal long-term brain damage.

    D. have permanent brain damage, if he can be resuscitated.

69. The 75-year-old woman suddenly clutches her chest and falls forward. She is now unresponsive. When assessing her breathing, you should **NOT**:

    A. lean over her nose and mouth to listen for breathing.

    B. watch for movement of her chest and abdomen.

    C. tap on both sides of her chest.

    D. feel for air movement against your face.

70. The 75-year-old woman is in cardiac arrest. You begin CPR, knowing that you should complete 10 cycles of 5:1 compressions and ventilations every:

    A. 15 to 20 seconds.

    B. 30 seconds or less.

    C. 40 to 53 seconds.

    D. 60 seconds.

Questions 71-76 refer to the information below.

A 20-year-old woman and her two young children, one aged 3 years and the other 9 months, have just been pulled from a burning building. The woman is conscious and alert, but both children are in cardiac arrest.

71. For the purposes of CPR, patients are classified as children according to their:

    A. age.

    B. weight.

    C. nutritional status.

    D. overall physical appearance.

Case Studies

72. Cardiac arrest in children is usually preceded by respiratory arrest, because children:

    A. consume oxygen two to three times faster than adults.

    B. often have long-term, chronic diseases.

    C. often have penetrating chest trauma.

    D. do not consume much oxygen due to their slower heart rate.

73. Chest compressions on the 3-year-old patient should be performed at a depth and rate of:

    A. 1/2" to 1", at a rate of 140/min.

    B. 1" to 1 1/2", at a rate of 100/min.

    C. 1" to 2", at a rate of 60 to 80/min.

    D. 3/4" to 2", at a rate of 100 to 120/min.

74. Chest compressions on the 9-month-old patient should be performed at a depth and rate of:

    A. 1/4" to 1/2", at a rate of 140/min.

    B. 1/2" to 1", at a rate of 100/min.

    C. 1" to 1 1/2", at a rate of 80 to 100/min.

    D. 1 1/2" to 2", at a rate of 100 to 120/min.

75. Your first attempt to ventilate the infant is unsuccessful. You should now:

    A. call an ALS unit and await their arrival.

    B. attempt to ventilate the patient with an adult bag-valve-mask device.

    C. perform chest compressions without ventilations.

    D. reposition the infant's head and then attempt to ventilate again.

Chapter 29

76. If you are still unable to ventilate the infant, you should next deliver:

    A. back blows until the airway is cleared.

    B. chest thrusts until the airway is cleared.

    C. five back blows and then five chest thrusts.

    D. four chest thrusts and then four back blows.

Questions 77-80 refer to the information below.

You are called to a local tavern for a "man down" and learn en route that the patient has been shot, but that law enforcement officials have the gunman in custody. Upon arrival, you see the patient lying at the foot of the front stairs leading into the tavern. A witness states that he saw the victim shot twice in the chest with a .38 special at point-blank range. On assessment, you see one entrance wound just below the left clavicle, and a second entrance wound just above the right nipple. There are two exit wounds in the patient's back that are in line with the entrance wounds.

77. The bullet that entered just below the left clavicle is **LEAST** likely to have hit which of the following structures?

    A. Aorta or the aortic arch

    B. Subclavian vein or artery

    C. A piece of the left lung

    D. Liver or the gallbladder

78. The entrance wound over the right nipple area bubbles each time the patient inhales. You should immediately:

    A. decompress the chest with a 14-gauge needle.

    B. apply a loose, sterile gauze dressing over the wound.

    C. apply an occlusive dressing over the wound.

    D. give oxygen via nasal cannula at 2 L/min.

Case Studies

79. The patient is having increasing difficulty breathing even though you are ventilating him with a bag-valve-mask device with 100% oxygen. His chest is hyperresonant, and his neck veins are distended. Breath sounds are absent on the right side. These signs and symptoms suggest a:

    A. tension pneumothorax.

    B. ruptured diaphragm.

    C. cardiac tamponade.

    D. massive hemothorax.

80. Given where you found the patient, you should begin:

    A. needle cricothyrotomy.

    B. transtracheal jet insufflation.

    C. full spinal immobilization.

    D. hypoventilation with a bag-valve-mask device.

Questions 81-84 refer to the information below.

You are called to a private residence for a "possible suicide." On arrival, you find a 23-year-old man unconscious and unresponsive sitting in the front seat of a car. The motor is running, and the garage door is nailed shut. You find empty beer cans and three or four empty pill bottles on the front seat of the car.

81. Your first step in this situation is to:

    A. check for a pulse.

    B. begin CPR.

    C. give oxygen via nasal cannula.

    D. move the patient to a safe environment.

82. The patient remains unconscious and unresponsive. Your primary concern for any patient in a coma is to:

    A. determine the cause.

    B. start an IV line.

    C. take baseline vital signs.

    D. protect the airway.

Chapter 29

83. Given the situation and the patient's unresponsiveness, you suspect:

    A. alcohol withdrawal syndrome.

    B. carbon monoxide poisoning.

    C. acute anaphylactic reaction.

    D. penetrating head trauma.

84. What information would be most useful to the medical control physician?

    A. Make and model of the car

    B. The patient's incontinence

    C. The patient's gender

    D. The name of the medications

Questions 85-87 refer to the information below.

A 76-year-old man has no pulse and is not breathing immediately after being pulled from a swimming pool. Your partner begins cardiac monitoring, but the rhythm on the monitor is indiscernable and full of artifact.

85. The artifact is most likely caused by:

    A. the age of the patient.

    B. a dead battery.

    C. patient movement.

    D. water on the skin.

86. The patient is in coarse ventricular fibrillation. To improve the chance for effective defibrillation, you should first:

    A. insert a properly sized oropharyngeal airway.

    B. place the patient prone on a flat, hard surface.

    C. apply special conductive defibrillation pads.

    D. apply and inflate a pneumatic antishock garment (PASG).

Case Studies

87. Just before defibrillating the patient, you should:

    A. begin CPR.

    B. begin an IV line with normal saline solution.

    C. confirm that no one is touching the patient.

    D. perform at least four back blows, followed by four chest thrusts.

Questions 88-92 refer to the information below.

You are called to an apartment building for a man who is "feeling ill." On arrival, you find a malnourished, middle-aged man lying on the couch who says he has been "vomiting for 2 days and his stomach hurts bad." He is very lethargic, and has pale, cool, slightly moist skin. He states that his wife left him about 6 months ago for a younger man and that he has been drinking "pretty heavy" since then. He has a blood pressure of 90/58 mm Hg, a pulse of 130/min, and respirations of 24/min.

88. Which of the following IV solutions would be most appropriate for this patient?

    A. 5% Dextrose

    B. 10% Dextrose

    C. 0.25 Normal saline solution

    D. Lactated Ringer's solution

89. What size catheter and administration set would be indicated?

    A. 14 gauge, with a mini-drip set

    B. 16 gauge, with a solution set

    C. 20 gauge, with a solution set

    D. 24 gauge, with a mini-drip set

90. Of the following IV sites, which best meet the patient's fluid replacement needs?

    A. Ventral hand

    B. Antecubital fossa

    C. Dorsal aspect of the hand

    D. Dorsal aspect of the foot

Chapter 29

91. After you prepare the site, and apply a tourniquet, you try to start the IV line. You get a flash back, but as you attempt to feed the catheter and withdraw the needle, the vein "blows," and a hematoma begins to form. You should:

    A. reinsert the needle into the catheter, withdraw them both, and apply pressure to the site for 1 to 2 minutes.

    B. reinsert the needle into the catheter, withdraw them both, and attempt a second IV line with a new catheter 1" to 2" below the original site.

    C. discard the needle in a sharps container, remove the catheter, and apply pressure to the site for 3 to 5 minutes.

    D. discard the needle in a sharps container, remove the catheter, and attempt a second IV line with a new catheter 3" to 5" below the original site.

92. After establishing the IV line, medical control orders you to administer 900 mL/hr. How fast would you set the flow rate if a 10 gtts/mL administration set is used? (Note: 1 mL = 1 cc)

    A. 150 gtts/min

    B. 90 gtts/min

    C. 15 gtts/min

    D. 10 gtts/min

Questions 93-95 apply to the information below:

A 62-year-old woman collapses with chest pain in the vegetable section of a grocery store. You find her sitting up and complaining of substernal chest pain that is radiating to her jaw. She states the pain started about 20 minutes ago when she was buying some corn. She has a blood pressure of 134/74 mm Hg, an irregular pulse of 102/min, and respirations of 18/min. The patient takes no medications, but is allergic to grapes and iodine.

93. Which of the following steps would **NOT** be appropriate before starting an IV in this patient?

    A. Assemble all the necessary equipment.

    B. Prepare the site with povoiodine and alcohol.

    C. Check the vein for a pulse.

    D. Apply an IV tourniquet 6" above the site.

364 Student Review Manual

Case Studies

94. The patient complains of pain at the site as you are starting the IV line, but says that she "feels better now." Your next step should be to:

    A. leave the catheter in place, and then reassure the patient.

    B. leave the catheter in place, and then rinse the site with alcohol.

    C. remove the catheter and apply pressure to the site for 3 to 5 minutes.

    D. remove the catheter and apply pressure to the site for 1 to 2 minutes.

95. The IV line has been running for 45 minutes when the patient begins to have difficulty breathing. She now has a blood pressure of 160/90 mm Hg, a pulse of 68/min, and respirations of 30/min. The patient's neck veins are distended, and you hear rales in both lungs. These signs and symptoms suggest:

    A. infection.

    B. anaphylaxis.

    C. overhydration.

    D. hypovolemia.

Questions 96-97 refer to the information below.

You are sent to a one-car rollover on a country road 15 minutes away. You find the car upside down in a drainage ditch, and first responders at the scene tell you to "hurry up" because they think the patient is going into shock. Immediately after the patient is extricated, you immediately apply an IV tourniquet and start the IV line in a large vein while your partner sets up the bag.

96. Given this situation and way in which the IV line was started, which of the following complications is most likely to develop?

    A. Infection

    B. Catheter shear

    C. Nerve damage

    D. Arterial puncture

Chapter 29

97. If the IV administration set is hooked up without flushing the tubing, which of the following complications could develop?

   A. Hematoma

   B. Air embolism

   C. Tissue slough

   D. Thrombophlebitis

Answers

1: **C.** In this situation, you must evaluate the patient's mental competency and ability to understand the consequences of his refusal. If the patient is not competent, which is not always an easy decision to make, then his refusal does not have any bearing on your decision to treat and/or transport. One of the grounds for a valid refusal of treatment is that the patient is mentally competent, and perhaps more importantly, able to understand the consequences of refusing treatment and transport. (ECTSI 5, p. 22)

2: **D.** Failure to continue treatment once you have begun to provide care constitutes abandonment. You must continue to provide care until responsibility is transferred to another health care professional of an equal or higher level of skill, or until the patient is transferred to a medical facility. Abandonment occurs when you stop treating a patient whom you have begun to treat (as in this situation), or turn the care of the patient over to someone less qualified, such as a paramedic leaving a patient to be transported by an EMT-A. (ECTSI 5, p. 23)

3: **A.** In order to leave this situation without the risk of being charged with abandonment, you and your partner needed to report and document that informed consent existed. The patient must not only expressly authorize treatment (actual consent) but must be mentally capable and must understand the type and extent of treatment, the consequences of a refusal of treatment, and any risks or possible complications associated with the treatment. (ECTSI 5, p. 21)

4: **C.** The term "Good Samaritan" comes from a biblical passage about a Samaritan who provides aid to an injured person whom he encounters along the roadway. Although Good Samaritan laws may provide immunity from liability, they do not prevent civil lawsuits from being filed, which can be very costly for the caregiver. (ECTSI 5, p. 24)

Case Studies

5: **D.** The most appropriate course of action in this situation is to contact medical control for instructions. Legally, you are the "on scene" extension of your service's medical director. In different jurisdictions this may be one physician per service, or one physician for several services, or a medical control committee that serves many squads or an entire city, county, or region. Regardless, it is the physician(s) whose signature(s) appear on the treatment protocols who have authorized you to perform certain procedures, not any physician who happens to arrive at the scene. (ECTSI 5, pp. 7–9)

6: **A.** The patient is coughing, which makes a certain degree of noise. Noise is produced by air passing through the vocal cords, and if noises are still present, at least a partial airway still remains. Great care must be taken to ensure that the patient's partial airway obstruction does not become a complete airway obstruction. As long as the patient can support herself, she is probably best able to clear the obstruction. You should remain by her side and encourage coughing and continued attempts by the patient to clear the obstruction. (ECTSI 5, p. 124)

7: **D.** The goal of the Heimlich maneuver is to attempt to "blow out" the obstruction from below. If the obstruction is not completely sealing the airway, it is likely that most of the pressurized air will simply escape from around the obstruction. In this situation, you should give the patient oxygen and provide prompt transport to the hospital for removal of the object. (ECTSI 5, p. 124)

8: **D.** Regardless of the drama and complexities of the rescue scene, your first responsibility is to make sure the scene is safe for you and your partner to enter to provide care. The fact that other workers and perhaps a rescue team is at the scene frantically working to extricate the patient does not mean that the scene is safe. (ECTSI 5, p. 46)

9: **D.** The patient's vital signs are considered borderline critical. Of the devices listed, only the nonrebreathing mask provides a high enough oxygen concentration to be of real benefit to this patient. (ECTSI 5, p. 182)

Chapter 29

10: **C.** The patient's breathing difficulties are due to constriction of the chest wall by the dirt surrounding him, not trauma. His continued efforts to breathe are producing fatigue in the intercostal muscles and actually reducing his ability to move the chest wall. At this point, you should provide active positive pressure ventilations with a bag-valve-mask device or demand valve to force high-concentration oxygen into his lungs. Both the Venturi mask and the nonrebreathing mask rely on the patient's ability to draw air into the lungs—an ability that is becoming more and more difficult for this patient. An emergency tracheostomy is not only beyond the level of training of an EMT-A, it would be of no benefit in this situation because the problem is below the level of the tracheostomy. (ECTSI 5, p. 184)

11: **A.** Blowing too fast or too vigorously can cause air to enter the esophagus rather than the trachea, which will cause inflation of the stomach (gastric distention) rather than the lungs. (ECTSI 5, p. 120)

12: **D.** With any unsuccessful ventilation attempt, you should first make sure that the patient's head and neck are in optimum position, and then try ventilating again. Given today's infection control standards, discarding the pocket mask to begin mouth-to-mouth breathing should not be considered unless there is definite equipment failure. Repositioning the head and slowing down the rate at which the ventilation is given should be your next move. (ECTSI 5, p. 131)

13: **D.** The first, most important step after determining that an adult patient is unresponsive is to activate the EMS system. You have already done this by telling a bystander to call 9-1-1. Your next step, then, is to open the patient's airway with the head-tilt/chin-lift maneuver and verify the absence of breathing with the look-listen-feel method. To complete the ABCs, you should next assess circulation by checking for a pulse and looking for major bleeding. (ECTSI 5, p. 110)

14: **D.** If the patient is not breathing, your next step is to provide two slow full mouth-to-mouth or mouth-to-mask ventilations. If the airway is open and the breaths go in, then check for a pulse. If the airway is obstructed and the breaths cannot be delivered, then begin proper care for an obstructed airway. (ECTSI 5, p. 117)

15: **A.** In this situation, although the patient appears to be dead, you must establish an open airway to begin CPR as soon as possible. (ECTSI 5, p. 111)

Case Studies

16: **B.** The position in which you found the patient would indicate that the patient's torso hit the steering wheel. While the other injuries listed may certainly be present, the internal chest injury is the only reliable choice from the information provided and is also consistent with producing enough damage to kill the patient quickly. (ECTSI 5, p. 224)

17: **C.** Even though the patient's injuries appear only minor, your primary concern is to find and/or rule out any obvious or hidden injuries that may be life threatening. Only after you have completed this step can you direct your attention to less serious problems. (ECTSI 5, p. 226)

18: **C.** It would be most helpful to know whether the child was able to walk and bear weight on his injured leg in determining the extent of musculoskeletal injury. The speed of the bicycle and the distance in which it skidded contribute to your knowledge about the severity of the mechanism of injury. Knowing how the child got to the porch will provide important information concerning loss of function. (ECTSI 5, p. 228)

19: **D.** All of the steps listed should be done before you begin caring for the patient. However, assessing motor function, sensation, and circulation in the injured leg should be done after a splint is applied. Reassessment will help to ensure that a nerve or blood vessel has not been injured as a result of the splint. A pulseless limb will die if circulation is not restored. (ECTSI 5, p. 271)

20: **C.** Shock is commonly a result of fluid or blood loss following an injury. When caused by blood loss, this type of shock is more specifically called hemorrhagic shock. (ECTSI 5, p. 210)

21: **B.** Applying direct pressure with your gloved hand, and soon thereafter (if not initially) with sterile dressings, is the first approach to controlling external bleeding. (ECTSI 5, p. 191)

22: **C.** Increasing intracranial pressure causes a pattern of vital signs that appears to be opposite that of a patient in shock. With increased intracranial pressure, the blood flow to the brain is reduced, resulting in increased hypoxia and cerebral edema. The body attempts to overcome this condition by slowing the pulse, improving cardiac output, and increasing blood pressure. (ECTSI 5, p. 329)

Chapter 29

23: **C.** Effective prehospital care for this patient is quite limited, as there is little you can really do in the prehospital setting for a closed head injury. However, with all head injuries, high-flow supplemental oxygen should be given to minimize hypoxia and possible cerebral edema. The brain requires a constant, rich supply of oxygen. Without it, severe brain damage or death may result in minutes. In this situation, a constant supply of oxygen will help to reduce blood levels of carbon dioxide and ultimately reduce intracranial pressure. (ECTSI 5, pp. 328–329)

24: **B.** The principal goal in immobilizing the patient's injury is to prevent motion of fracture fragments, a dislocated joint, or damaged soft tissues, thus reducing pain. Splinting also helps with transporting the patient. In a suspected fracture of the shaft of any bone, make sure the splint immobilizes the joint above and below the fracture. With injuries in and around the joint, make sure the splint immobilizes the bone above and the bone below the injured joint. In effect, you should expect to fully immobilize the entire extremity whenever a patient has an extremity injury. (ECTSI 5, p. 275)

25: **B.** In this situation, a sling and swathe is the best choice for immobilizing the extremity. The sling will support the weight of the arm and relieve the downward pull of gravity on the injury site. The swathe will prevent the humerus from moving away from the body and irritating the joint. (ECTSI 5, p. 287)

26: **C.** The shoulder girdle is composed of the clavicle anteriorly, the scapula posteriorly, and the upper end of the humerus laterally. The tibia is a bone of the lower leg. (ECTSI 5, p. 61)

27: **C.** The location of the patient's deformity is consistent with an anterior dislocation of the humeral head. The humeral head almost always dislocates anteriorly, coming to lie in front of the scapula. (ECTSI 5, p. 288)

28: **D.** A properly applied sling and swathe will provide support under the arm to help reduce pain caused by gravity pulling the arm down. You can stabilize the arm by placing a pillow or rolled blanket between the arm and the chest wall to fill up the space between them. Once the arm is stabilized, you can apply the sling and secure the pillow and sling with a swathe. (ECTSI 5, p. 289)

29: **B.** Assessment of distal circulation may be accomplished by checking the pulse, the color, temperature, and moisture of the skin, and capillary refill. Because assessing the patient's radial pulse causes so much pain, try one of these other methods for checking circulatory status. (ECTSI 5, pp. 80–81)

Case Studies

30: **A.** Immobilization of the hand and wrist in "the position of function," with the wrist slightly dorsiflexed and all finger joints moderately flexed, can help to reduce the possibility of later disability. (ECTSI 5, p. 296)

31: **B.** The initial goal of stabilizing the lower radius/ulna and wrist area requires immobilizing the elbow. Therefore, the radius, humerus, and metacarpals must be splinted. The fibula and femur are bones in the leg. (ECTSI 5, p. 295)

32: **A.** The patient's vital signs are within normal limits, with slightly elevated pulse and respirations due to the anxiety surrounding the injury. Compensated shock is characterized by elevated pulse and respirations; decompensated shock is characterized by decreased blood pressure. (ECTSI 5, p. 212)

33: **B.** This situation is probably ideal for using a pillow splint because the patient's injured hand will very likely swell. A pillow splint can surround the injured area firmly yet will yield inward and not create undue pressure when the injured area swells. In this cold-weather situation, the air splint may not provide reliable pressure and may, in fact, become too tight if the patient's hand begins to swell. (ECTSI 5, pp. 277–278)

34: **D.** The patient's increased pulse and respirations, changes in skin color, and decreased blood pressure suggest decompensated shock. (ECTSI 5, p. 212)

35: **C.** Hypovolemic shock, specifically hemorrhagic shock, is most consistent with the patient's vital signs and mechanism of injury. The patient does not have any visible bleeding; therefore, external bleeding would not be the cause of the shock. (ECTSI 5, p. 210)

36: **C.** The deformity of the thigh suggests a possible fractured femur. The strong signs of shock suggest that the bone ends have overridden and caused a capsule to form in which blood is collecting. (ECTSI 5, p. 304)

37: **D.** The patient has an open fracture, and as such, your first step in treatment is to control bleeding and limit possible contamination of the wound. After the bleeding is addressed, you may then begin measures to immobilize the extremity. (ECTSI 5, p. 274)

Chapter 29

38: **D.** Once applied, traction must not be released or lost. Therefore, you and your partner must maintain traction as the loops of the ankle hitch are connected to the end of the splint. (ECTSI 5, p. 280)

39: **C.** Place the ankle hitch about the foot first and then apply traction with your hands. Apply only enough traction to align the limb so that it will fit into the splint. Traction should be maintained while the ankle hitch is connected to the end of the splint. Placing the ankle hitch around the foot and ankle first allows either you or your partner (whoever is the lead EMT in applying the splint) to connect the ratchet mechanism without moving your hands to install the ankle hitch. (ECTSI 5, p. 280)

40: **D.** Given the patient's statements and the mechanism of injury, you should prepare to care for possible spinal cord injury. Pain and a tingling sensation are signs consistent with some type of spinal cord damage. A patient who has a severed spinal cord would not be able to stand or move; therefore, of the choices listed, swelling and/or pressure on the spinal cord is the most likely injury. (ECTSI 5, pp. 338–339)

41: **D.** The fact that the patient is standing indicates that the spinal cord has not been severed yet. Spinal immobilization is absolutely necessary given the mechanism of injury and the patient's complaints about pain and tingling. Because you do not know the extent of the spinal injury, you must take every precaution with the spine to prevent additional injury. (ECTSI 5, p. 339)

42: **D.** The proper way to prepare the patient for transport would be to fully immobilize him on a long spine board while he is still standing and then lower the board onto the stretcher. Once you suspect a spinal injury, make all efforts to avoid damage to the spinal cord. Any extraordinary motion (such as walking or sitting down), even as little as 1 mm, may cause significant spinal cord injury. (ECTSI 5, pp. 342–343)

43: **D.** With police, fire, and rescue services already "functioning" at the scene, the duties of the EMTs should focus on patient care only. While the EMT team has overall responsibility for the patient's well-being, the team would not assume the responsibilities of the other services, unless the team is asked to help. (ECTSI 5, p. 702)

44: **D.** Incident command should be in place in this situation; therefore, your first responsibility at the scene is to identify the leader or incident commander and coordinate your team's efforts with the incident commander. If a less formal structure exists, you should still attempt to determine who is in charge and then coordinate your team's efforts with the leader. (ECTSI 5, p. 702)

Case Studies

45: **A.** Unless you have already been advised that the injuries are minor and that only one ambulance is needed, it would be wise to call for more help as soon as possible. Unnecessary ambulances can always be sent back, but unnecessary delays while waiting for more help can have devastating results. (ECTSI 5, p. 703)

46: **D.** The patient's current condition suggests a pneumothorax that has progressed to a tension pneumothorax. The traumatic injury sealed with an occlusive dressing confirms the picture. (ECTSI 5, pp. 380–381)

47: **D.** Pneumothorax occurs as a result of air leaking into the pleural space from an opening in the chest wall or the lung. Hemothorax is the presence of blood in the chest cavity within the pleural space. Hemothorax and pneumothorax often coexist; both of these conditions are the result of the chest cavity becoming filled with something other than the lungs. (ECTSI 5, pp. 381–382)

48: **C.** Immediate treatment should include releasing one corner of the occlusive dressing to release the accumulated air. Oftentimes simply releasing the dressing is effective in relieving the problem. The air accumulated under pressure in the pleural space will rush from the wound once the dressing is released. (ECTSI 5, p. 381)

49: **C.** Before beginning any patient assessment or management, you must assess the scene for any hazards to the rescue team or the patient. Your first step in this situation would be to call the utility company to shut off the power. (ECTSI 5, p. 606)

50: **A.** Asystole is the proper term to describe total absence of electrical activity of the heart. It is represented by a straight line on the cardiac monitor. (ECTSI 5, p. 820)

51: **C.** The longer the patient remains in ventricular fibrillation, the less likely it is that he or she can be resuscitated. Given that the patient is already in fine ventricular fibrillation, he has most likely been fibrillating for some time, and will need to be shocked as soon as possible. (ECTSI 5, pp. 159–160)

52: **A.** Standing orders are designed to expedite patient care, especially under specific circumstances where a delay in care would cause further harm to the patient. (ECTSI 5, p. 823)

53: **C.** Opening the airway is critical, especially in this situation because the patient still has a pulse. The sooner the airway is open and secure, and oxygen is administered, the greater the chance that the patient will not go into cardiac arrest. (ECTSI 5, p. 709)

Chapter 29

54: **A.** The patient's signs and symptoms represent the classic presentation of a crush injury that in turn produces traumatic asphyxia. (ECTSI 5, p. 379)

55: **C.** Pressure over the cricoid member, the Sellick maneuver, is a technique used to occlude the esophagus and reduce the chance of vomiting during an intubation attempt. (ECTSI 5, p. 801)

56: **D.** If an endotracheal tube is inserted too far, it will often follow the angle of the right main stem bronchus, which will leave the patient's left lung unventilated. As a result, there will be no breath sounds when you auscultate the left side of the chest. The endotracheal tube should then be withdrawn 1" and the position checked again by listening for bilateral breath sounds. (ECTSI 5, p. 801)

57: **D.** Even though you are at a park at a family picnic, you should not assume that the scene is safe, as a family disturbance could have occurred. Ensuring the safety of the scene is your first responsibility. (ECTSI 5, p. 12)

58: **B.** The patient appears to be in cardiac arrest, but you should first assess the patient's level of consciousness (responsiveness), according to the 1992 AHA standards for adult one-rescuer CPR. (ECTSI 5, p. 112)

59: **B.** Even though the collapse was witnessed by several people, the fact that no BLS measures were provided decreases the patient's chance of survival. (ECTSI 5, p. 111)

60: **D.** You must first remove the child from the pool for effective resuscitation to take place. (ECTSI 5, p. 636)

61: **C.** Even though it is unlikely that a 2-year-old child was diving when this accident occurred, the possibility of a cervical spine injury still exists. Therefore, the jaw-thrust technique would be the most appropriate way to open the patient's airway. (ECTSI 5, pp. 125, 637)

62: **A.** Since the patient still has a pulse, she is in respiratory arrest at this point and only needs artificial ventilation followed by oxygen therapy. (ECTSI 5, pp. 124–125)

63: **A.** The physical appearance of this patient is consistent with livor mortis or dependent lividity. This condition suggests that an extended time has passed since the patient died. (ECTSI 5, p. 78)

Case Studies

64: **D.** Starting CPR on a person who has been dead long enough for the body to show the signs of livor mortis, or dependent lividity, is not necessary. (ECTSI 5, p. 79)

65: **B.** The cool, dry skin, and the purplish discoloration on the patient's back and buttocks are significant factors to consider with regard to your decision about whether or not to begin a resuscitation attempt. (ECTSI 5, pp. 78–79)

66: **B.** Both women are obviously alive, and in all probability in less critical condition than the patient who is lying supine and is cyanotic and possibly in cardiac arrest. (ECTSI 5, p. 608)

67: **B.** Due to its size and close proximity to the central circulation, the carotid artery would be the best pulse to check on any of these patients. (ECTSI 5, p. 145)

68: **D.** If 10 minutes have elapsed since the patient went into cardiac arrest, he is well outside the normal 4- to 6-minute window where resuscitation is likely to save the patient and result in little or no neurologic deficit. Permanent brain damage is very likely, if the patient can be resuscitated. (ECTSI 5, p. 110)

69: **C.** Looking, listening, and feeling for the signs of air movement would be a more valuable BLS respiratory assessment than percussing or tapping the chest. (ECTSI 5, p. 117)

70: **D.** According to the 1992 AHA standards for adult one-rescuer CPR, 10 cycles of 15:2 compressions every minute. (ECTSI 5, p. 148)

71: **A.** Any patient between the ages of 1 and 8 years is considered a child by AHA standards. (ECTSI 5, p. 151)

72: **A.** Since children consume oxygen two to three times faster than adults, cardiac arrest is usually secondary to hypoxia and myocardial ischemia. (ECTSI 5, p. 151)

73: **B.** According to the 1992 AHA standards for child CPR, the chest should be compressed 1" to 1 1/2", at a rate of 100/min. (ECTSI 5, p. 153)

74: **B.** According to the 1992 AHA standards for infant CPR, the chest should be compressed 1/2" to 1", at a rate of at least 100/min. (ECTSI 5, pp. 152–153)

Chapter 29

75: **D.** If your first attempt to ventilate the patient is unsuccessful, you should reposition the head and attempt to ventilate again, before trying other BLS interventions. (ECTSI 5, p. 126)

76: **C.** If you are unable to ventilate an infant after one attempt, repositioning the head, and then trying for a second time, you should deliver five back blows, followed by five chest thrusts. (ECTSI 5, p. 127)

77: **D.** Because there is an exit wound behind the entrance wound, this bullet would not hit organs located in the right upper quadrant of the abdominal cavity. However, the other answer choices listed are all possibilities. (ECTSI 5, p. 391)

78: **C.** All open chest wounds should be sealed, especially wounds large enough to allow air to be sucked into the chest cavity. Over a period of time, a tension pneumothorax could possibly develop when such a wound has been sealed. Therefore, you should periodically monitor for signs of a developing tension pneumothorax. (ECTSI 5, pp. 382–383)

79: **A.** The patient's signs and symptoms are consistent with a tension pneumothorax. As the pressure in the chest rises, blood flow to the heart diminishes, cardiac output drops, and the patient gets progressively worse. If not treated, the patient will die. (ECTSI 5, p. 380)

80: **C.** The patient was found at the bottom of a flight of stairs, which means he could have fallen without taking steps to break or soften his fall. This mechanism of injury could produce a spinal injury. (ECTSI 5, p. 337)

81: **D.** Even though you can stop the car, the fact that the garage door is nailed shut prevents you from providing adequate ventilation for the patient. Therefore, the patient must be moved to a location where he can be safely cared for without putting the rescue team at risk. (ECTSI 5, p. 602)

82: **D.** Establishing and maintaining a patent airway is the top priority for this patient. (ECTSI 5, p. 602)

83: **B.** A known suicide attempt in which the patient is in a running automobile suggests carbon monoxide poisoning. (ECTSI 5, p. 602)

84: **D.** Even though carbon monoxide poisoning is a key concern, determining what medications may have been ingested is also important. Drug overdose could hamper any resuscitation efforts. (ECTSI 5, p. 664)

Case Studies

85: **D.** Good skin contact is important for monitoring electrodes. A hairy or moist chest and/or dry electrodes are three very common reasons that excessive artifact often appears on the monitor. (ECTSI 5, p. 826)

86: **C.** Use of special defibrillation pads or gel is designed to reduce resistance to the current and improve penetration, thus improving the chances for a successful defibrillation. (ECTSI 5, p. 823)

87: **C.** The person operating the defibrillator is responsible for ensuring that no member of the rescue team, including himself or herself, is in contact with the patient during the delivery of the electrical countershock. (ECTSI 5, p. 825)

88: **D.** Lactated Ringer's solution would be most appropriate for this patient since he has been vomiting for 2 days and is showing signs of shock. Lactated Ringer's solution, with its composition of electrolytes, would be the fluid of choice. (ECTSI 5, p. 784)

89: **B.** When fluid replacement is indicated, the largest, shortest catheter possible should be used in conjunction with a solution set. While a 14-gauge catheter is the largest, it is paired with the wrong administration set. (ECTSI 5, pp. 785–786)

90: **B.** Of the choices listed, the antecubital fossa would provide the largest veins, allowing more volume to be administered. The other sites listed have smaller veins. (ECTSI 5, p. 787)

91: **C.** Once a needle has been removed from a catheter, it should not be reinserted for any reason, as it increases the likelihood of a catheter shear. Second attempts should be done in another extremity, or if in the same extremity, proximal to the original site. (ECTSI 5, p. 790)

92: **A.** The order is for 900 mL/hr or 15 mL/min using an administration set. An administration set that delivers 1 mL for every 10 drops results in a flow rate of 150 gtts/min. (ECTSI 5, p. 790)

93: **B.** The patient states she is allergic to iodine; therefore, you should not use povoiodine. Use alcohol only. (ECTSI 5, pp. 787–788)

94: **A.** Pain during the actual IV attempt is normal. However, the pain should quickly subside after the IV line is in place. If pain continues, the IV line may have infiltrated and would then need to be removed. (ECTSI 5, p. 790)

Chapter 29

95: **C.** The patient's signs and symptoms indicate that the patient has received too much fluid too quickly. The IV line should be shut down and removed, or if it is absolutely necessary to maintain IV access, it should be slowed to a TKO rate (6 to 8 gtts/min). (ECTSI 5, p. 791)

96: **A.** Starting an IV line in the field is difficult enough because of the uncontrolled setting. You should be especially careful to properly prepare the site before starting the IV line because of the many "dirty environments" in which patients are found. Failure to properly prepare the site before initiating the IV line greatly increases the likelihood of infection. (ECTSI 5, p. 791)

97: **B.** Failure to flush the IV tubing could result in an air embolism. (ECTSI 5, p. 791)